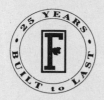

LIVING WITH TOURETTE SYNDROME

Elaine Fantle Shimberg

A FIRESIDE BOOK
PUBLISHED BY SIMON & SCHUSTER
New York   London   Toronto   Sydney   Tokyo   Singapore

FIRESIDE
Rockefeller Center
1230 Avenue of the Americas
New York, NY 10020

Designed by Irving Perkins Associates

Manufactured in the United States of America

10 9 8 7 6 5 4

Library of Congress Cataloging-in-Publication Data
Shimberg, Elaine Fantle, 1937–
    Living with Tourette syndrome / Elaine Fantle Shimberg.
        p.   cm.
    "A Fireside book."
    Includes bibliographical references and index.
    1. Tourette syndrome—Popular works.   I. Title.
    RC375.S55   1995
    362.1'9683—dc20   95-20038
                                                 CIP

ISBN 0-684-81160-X

Grateful acknowledgment is made to the following sources for permission to reprint
material in their control:

Excerpt from *Arthritis on the Job: You Can Work with It,* © 1994 by the Arthritis
Foundation. Reprinted with permission of the Arthritis Foundation. For further
information or for a complete copy of this booklet, write to the Arthritis
Foundation, P.O. Box 19000, Atlanta, GA 30326, or contact your local Arthritis
Foundation chapter.
    Some of the materials in Chapter 15 were adapted from the author's previous
works, *Strokes: What Families Should Know,* and *Depression: What Families
Should Know,* published by Ballantine Books.
    Excerpt from *Driven to Distraction* by Edward M. Hallowell, M.D., and John J.
Ratey, M.D., © 1994 by Edward M. Hallowell, M.D., and John J. Ratey, M.D.
Reprinted by permission of Pantheon Books, a division of Random House, Inc.
    Excerpt from *American Psychiatric Association: Diagnostic and Statistical
Manual of Mental Disorders, Fourth Edition.* © 1994 by American Psychiatric
Association. Reprinted with permission.

The information contained in this book reflects the author's experience, research,
and interviews with others and is in no way intended to replace competent medical,
legal, or other professional advice. Specific medical opinions can be given only by
qualified physicians, specially trained psychologists, social workers, and others in
the health-care field who are familiar with Tourette Syndrome and its symptoms,
and are aware of each person's particular medical history and other relevant
information.
    Always consult your doctor.

Acknowledgments

No book, especially one of this scope, is ever the effort of just one person. There are many people who contributed in countless ways. However, without the interest, cooperation, and encouragement of two very special women, this book never would have been written. I am forever indebted to them—Faith Hamlin, my agent, and Sue Levi-Pearl, medical liaison of the Tourette Syndrome Association and friend. Thank you, thank you, thank you.

Special thanks also to my supportive editor, Sheila M. Curry, and to my wonderful medical and educational advisory panel— Rosa A. Hagin, Ph.D.; Ruth D. Bruun, M.D.; Christopher Goetz, M.D.; Roger Freeman, M.D.; the late Arthur Shapiro, M.D.; Elaine Shapiro, Ph.D.; Jacqueline Favish, M.Ed.; and Sue Levi-Pearl—all of whom spent some of their precious summer hours reviewing the manuscript for accuracy. Their detailed comments and suggested additions (and deletions) demonstrated their support and desire to make this book one that they could comfortably recommend.

I especially appreciated the parents, spouses, and individuals with Tourette Syndrome who freely expressed their thoughts, fears, and frustrations in dealing with TS. Thanks, too, to Lois Linet, Alan Levitt, Joseph Jankovic, M.D., Sue Wiggins, Archie Silver, M.D., Susan Conners, Ramona Fisher Collins, Jean Valencia, Mort Doran, M.D., Emily Kelman-Bravo, CSW, MS, and numerous others.

The entire staff of the Tourette Syndrome Association were extremely supportive in either answering my questions or finding someone who could. They never once hinted that I was interrupting their own work. I owe them all a tremendous debt of gratitude.

Special thanks to all who shared their "Success Stories" and permitted me to retell them, using their real names. Lastly, love and thanks to my own family, for once again agreeing to let me use our personal lives as a canvas on which to paint a tale.

Dedicated to Judie Taggart Rhodin

Who succeeded doing in one day
what took me thirty years to accomplish.

Contents

PART IV: SCHOOL ISSUES

PART V: ADULT ISSUES

Author's Note

In the years since my children were diagnosed with Tourette Syndrome, I have written numerous books on medical subjects including irritable bowel syndrome, strokes, depression, and brain stem and spinal cord disorders in children. Yet, other than a handful of articles for major magazines and a booklet for the Tourette Syndrome Association, "Coping with Tourette Syndrome: A Parent's Viewpoint," written in 1979 and revised in 1994, I have not written on Tourette Syndrome. Why, I wondered?

I think the answer is that, as my children grew out of their teens and into adulthood, their tics either became very minimal or completely disappeared, as often happens. With that subconscious protection called denial, I disavowed that anything had ever been wrong. "It's not part of my life anymore," I convinced my inner self and put a distance between myself and TS.

Then, two things happened that forced me to examine my viewpoint. After completing the book *Gifts of Time* with Dr. Fred J. Epstein, my agent, Faith Hamlin, asked what other medical subjects I might like to tackle for my next book. I gave her a list of ten. Tourette Syndrome was number ten.

"What is it?" she asked. "And how do you know about it?" I explained. "What books are out there for the layperson?" she probed.

"Not a great many," I admitted. But I confessed that I wasn't sure that there was much of a need.

I went home, mulling over the possibility of doing a book on TS. I wasn't sure I wanted to do it. I mentioned it to a pediatrician I knew slightly.

"I have two patients with mild TS," he said. "It isn't full-blown because they don't curse. I told one youngster that he was hurting his parents with all those noises and movements and that he should cut it out. I gave his parents permission to kick him in the pants when he made those sounds.''

"But coprolalia isn't required to make a diagnosis of TS," I said carefully. "And if it is Tourette Syndrome, he can't help making those movements and sounds. It's neurological, not psychological.''

"That's why I called it 'not full-blown,' " the doctor responded, obviously not wanting to continue our conversation.

For two days, I thought about a little boy being spanked because of his tics. Then I called my agent. "Let's do it," I said. "I want to write a book about Tourette Syndrome.''

This book is for families and friends of those with TS, for physicians and other health-care professionals who want and need to know more about this baffling disorder, and for teachers, administrators, coaches, guidance counselors, school nurses, and all the others who deal with TS in the academic world.

Introduction

We were fortunate in the early years of our study of Tourette Syndrome (TS) to meet the Shimbergs. Those of us who do research, treat and advise patients always owe a debt of gratitude to those who valiantly struggle with their affliction because they provide us with an in-depth understanding of the disorder, sensitivity to its effects, and respect for those so afflicted. The Shimberg family did all of this and much more. TS at the time was considered a rare illness and funding agencies were unwilling to grant funds until they knew there were sufficient patients to provide an adequate sample for study. Fortunately for us, the Shimbergs had no such qualms. Challenged, as we were, by the need to understand and treat TS, they supported our research without hesitation, and provided encouragement, support, friendship, and continued loyalty. Their support contributed to achieving greater knowledge about the diagnosis, nosology, epidemiology, and treatment of TS. The avalanche of knowledge and information on TS makes the present volume particularly relevant today. We feel honored, therefore, to write an introduction to this informative book on TS.

Living with Tourette Syndrome, the subject of Elaine Fantle Shimberg's book, clearly testifies to her understanding as a layperson of this complex disorder. She has written a comprehensive book providing information about the diagnosis, treatment, genetics, and other putative causative factors. It is also an excellent primer for patients, parents, and teachers about the difficulties of daily life: how to cope with the illness in the family, in school, at work, as a teen, as an adult, and the agencies and organizations to turn to for help. The book is unique in providing this essential information in an easy-to-read, informative, sensitively written, and caring way. Interspersed throughout are comments about her own experience as a sufferer, mother of three children with TS, wife, and writer. She has written this book from a comprehensive perspective and has done it well.

Living with Tourette Syndrome focuses on the most difficult patients because they are the ones usually taken to the doctor, research center, or agency for evaluation and therefore labeled as "patients." Such patients frequently have more severe symptoms and may have, as the author refers to them, "tagalong" illnesses. They are apt to experience greater difficulties in coping and they and their families often require advice and help in managing all aspects of their illness and lives. At the same time, Shimberg acknowledges that many individuals have mild symptoms and most do not seek any medical help because their tics do not interfere with their functioning. This, in fact, represents our own experience and research with this disorder. We found that the majority of patients have mild symptoms, cope well with their illness, respond well to medication at low dosages, and do not have associated attention deficit hyperactivity disorder (ADHD), obsessive-compulsive disorder (OCD), or other psychological problems. These controversies about the relationship of ADHD and OCD to TS and its treatment are also acknowledged by the author.

She includes an interesting and uplifting chapter entitled "Celebrating Success Stories." An author, of necessity, must be reticent about celebrating his or her own success. Fortunately, we are not subject to the same reticence. This book provides ample evidence of Shimberg's successful struggle to deal with her own illness, her empathy, compassion, and support for her children with TS—indeed for everyone's children—and her unstinting work with parents, doctors, schools, and organizations to educate them about TS.

We firmly believe that *Living with Tourette Syndrome* is an invaluable source book and will contribute to easing the burden of patients and their families.

—Arthur K. Shapiro, M.D., LFAPA
Clinical Professor of Psychiatry

—Elaine Shapiro, Ph.D.
Associate Professor of Psychiatry

Mount Sinai School of Medicine

Part I

CHAPTER 1

Remembering

When I was eight years old I wiggled my nose. Like a rabbit. I sniffed and I blinked too.

"Don't do that," my mother commanded.

"I can't help it," I answered.

"Curl your toes instead," she said. "That way no one will see you."

So I curled my toes inside my shoes whenever I felt like wiggling my nose, or sniffing or blinking. And eventually—I don't remember when—I stopped doing that, too.

I had Tourette Syndrome and nobody knew. Until I had children. . . .

CHAPTER 2

Revisited[1]

Like all new mothers, I counted my baby's tiny fingers and toes as soon as she was placed in my arms, as though having the proper number of digits guaranteed that she was (and the unspoken covenant was that she would continue to be) "all right." Indeed, she was blessed with ten miniature fingers and ten tiny toes. Innocent as I was, I relaxed my vigilance, relieved to know that my baby was "perfect."

In rapid order, we added to our family. Fifteen months later we had a son. A second daughter was born twenty-one months after him, and in another thirteen months, our second son.

We were a busy and happy family. The children were well behaved and fun. Our photo albums quickly filled with pictures of our travels with the brood to dude ranches, resorts, cities, and various tourist attractions. We took them out for regular family Sunday night dinners and to movies, theater, and sporting events. We were the fortunate ones, we said thankfully. We had been truly blessed with bright and healthy children. When our youngest was almost four, we decided to have another baby. I quickly became pregnant with our fifth child.

Then, our lives changed. I had often reminded our children that anyone can be happy, outgoing, and upbeat when fortune smiles,

---

[1] Parts of this chapter have been adapted from writings by this author, which first appeared in the book *Gilles de la Tourette Syndrome* by Arthur K. Shapiro, Elaine S. Shapiro, Ruth D. Bruun, and Richard D. Sweet, published by Raven Press, New York City, in 1978.

but that the true mark of a person's character is how he or she handles adversity. We were about to experience that firsthand.

When did my oldest child's symptoms begin? Who knows? One day we simply became aware that our seven-year-old little girl was doing "it" again. "It" was just a shrug of her shoulders. Nothing more. But wait . . . soon it became a shrug combined with a neck jerk, as though she had a crick in her neck. And it seemed to happen not once, but constantly. She began to complain that her neck ached.

We took her to our pediatrician, a kindly old man who had always known the answers. Like most laypeople, we felt he knew everything necessary to care for our child. He gave her a complete checkup and assured us that it was, no doubt, a "simple childhood tic" that would go away shortly.

Reassured, we pretended to ignore it. And we ignored the way she was beginning to blink . . . and sniff . . . and clear her throat. Frightened, we didn't speak of it to one another. "Ignore it," we had been advised. Neither of us wanted to confess to the other that we couldn't ignore it.

Our daughter called the tics her "habit." But she wondered why she couldn't control the motions or silence the sounds. Now her arms were jerking too, as though some unseen puppet master was jerking invisible strings. I wanted to cradle her in my arms, to "kiss it away," do anything to stop it. Never have I felt so helpless. I wondered if we were being too strict, too permissive, or too . . . what? Was she upset over this pregnancy? School problems? Well-meaning friends and extended family offered their opinions: She watched too much television . . . wasn't getting enough sleep . . . was seeking more attention.

"I can't help it," she'd cry.

"She can't help it," we'd echo, defending her to the world, and yet all the while wondering to ourselves what terrible demons were attacking her. Was it possible that she *was* emotionally disturbed, we whispered to each other in the dark. We couldn't believe that. Other than the tics, she seemed perfectly normal to us. However, we knew about parental denial. Perhaps she *did* have mental problems. Then, and for no apparent reason, the sniffing and throat clearing stopped.

But before we had time to be thankful and heave a sigh of relief, those tics were replaced by hooting, and then barking sounds. It was too painful to continue to do nothing. We made an appointment with a pediatric neurologist.

"I think it's just a bad habit. She'll outgrow it during puberty," he intoned, plucking at the hairs in his beard. "Don't worry about it unless it becomes debilitating."

But what *is* debilitating? Is it when your child's arm shoots out, spilling the contents of her glass all over the table? Is it when her chest throbs with pain at night because she exhales so violently with each hooting sound? Is it when she chokes on her food because her tongue darts out while she's eating?

Where were the experts? Where were the medical people we had always counted on to give us the answers? Where was help? We felt desperately frustrated, bewildered, and so alone.

There were more appointments with doctors—another neurologist, a psychiatrist, and then a very young psychologist just beginning his practice. He had trained with a doctor who had treated a few patients with the same symptoms as our daughter.

"I don't think she has 'childhood tics,' " he said. "I think she has something called Tourette Syndrome."

It was the first time we had ever heard the term.

He talked about the possibility of using a powerful drug, called haloperidol (Haldol). Then he mentioned its side effects. They were frightening. He admitted that he didn't know any psychiatrist or neurologist locally with experience in using it to treat Tourette Syndrome. After much agonizing, we decided to try his alternative suggestion—that of behavior modification.

For three months, five days a week, we took our then ten-year-old daughter to the psychologist. Her throat ached from producing the bizarre barking sounds over and over again. My heart ached from watching her and agonizing over whether this type of treatment could really help.

It seemed to be effective. The sounds did go away and we rejoiced. Little did we know that this was simply part of the waxing and waning pattern of her disorder. We were so encouraged . . . only to be bitterly disappointed one month later when the symptoms returned and were even worse than before. Our child considered it a personal failure. When we returned to see the psychologist, she turned her chair away so that she didn't have to face him.

Now she was twelve. Five painful years had crept by as we tried to make some sense out of what was happening. The uncertainty of it all was overwhelming, preoccupying our every waking moment, disturbing our dreams.

Then fate stepped in. While sitting in a doctor's waiting room, I happened upon a brief paragraph in a weekly news magazine, describing a man with tics similar to those our daughter was displaying. It mentioned a psychiatrist, Dr. Arthur Shapiro, who practiced in New York City and was treating this man and others who had a disorder known as Tourette Syndrome. That day we made plans to fly with our daughter to New York and Dr. Shapiro.

After examining her and taking a careful history, the doctor confirmed that she, indeed, was showing the classic symptoms of the neurological disorder known as Tourette Syndrome.

At last we knew without doubt what was wrong. Our little girl wasn't crazy or nervous, wasn't acting out jealousy, resentment, or anger. She wasn't trying for attention or any of the other scenarios suggested by the other professionals we had seen. I wasn't a bad or overbearing mother. Our daughter had something physical—an imbalance in the neurotransmitters of her brain, the chemicals controlling movement and verbal actions. Her tics were involuntary. She had Tourette Syndrome.

A few years later, we learned that two of our other children also had Tourette Syndrome. But knowing what it was gave us all the strength to cope. It had been the unknown, the terror of the shadows, that had tormented us the most.

This is why I have chosen to write *Living with Tourette Syndrome*—in the hope that others won't have to walk those darkened streets alone.

It had taken us five exhausting years to learn what was wrong with our daughter. But our story is no different from hundreds of others. Although it all happened more than twenty years ago, even today, in most areas the typical person with Tourette Syndrome is usually seen by a minimum of four or five professionals before receiving a correct diagnosis, often spending years in expensive and time-consuming psychotherapy wondering if he or she is crazy. Says Dr. Shapiro, ''The burden of patients with Tourette Syndrome is so immense, it is a wonder to us and a credit to them that they do not become psychotic.''

Part II

WHAT *IS* TOURETTE SYNDROME?

CHAPTER 3

Learning the Symptoms

When my daughter was diagnosed with Tourette Syndrome in 1974, it was the first time any of us had ever heard the term. Back in the early seventies, TS was considered to be an extremely rare disorder, one so uncommon that most of the physicians I then discussed it with were as unfamiliar with the disorder as we were. Those who did recognize the name vaguely recalled reading a paragraph or two about it in some medical text that described Tourette Syndrome as some type of a rare tic disorder, but they apologetically admitted that they didn't know much about it.

Some thought it was a psychological disorder, and many others referred to it as "that cursing disease." Usually, however, we got blank looks from the health-care professionals—pediatricians, neurologists, psychologists, and psychiatrists—that one normally sees when a child begins to have verbal and motor tics.

Today, thanks primarily to the efforts of the Tourette Syndrome Association and its dedicated professional and lay volunteers, a larger proportion of the medical community and lay population has at least heard of TS, although they may not be aware of all its many variations and complexities.

In the scientific literature, TS is often referred to as "Gilles de la Tourette's Syndrome," named for the French physician who first suggested in 1885 that the symptoms were part of a distinct condition different from other movement disorders. It is also called *Tourette's disorder* and *Tourette Syndrome*. I prefer the latter term and it is the one used throughout this book.

Tourette Syndrome is a chronic neurobiological tic disorder involving both motor and phonic tics. It is *not* (as formerly was thought) a psychological illness or psychosis nor is it an "acting out" of resentments, frustrations, or anger; it is not a nervous habit nor is it a means of getting attention. It is biochemically based and, in most cases, genetically transmitted, although there are some case histories of individuals developing Tourette Syndrome after suffering neonatal brain damage or other trauma to the brain or without known family history.

What It Looks and Sounds Like

To the uninitiated, seeing someone with obvious and severe Tourette Syndrome for the first time is often a baffling, bizarre, and yet fascinating experience. There's a split second of confusion. "Did I see it or didn't I?" You want to look away, not stare, but you're too curious to see what might happen next. On the one hand, the constant multiple physical gyrations—such as head jerking, arms flailing, blinking, touching, tongue thrusting—and numerous nonsensical vocalizations—including grunts, hisses, squeaks, sniffing, barks, and hoots—resemble the antics of what we stereotypically consider to be those of a "crazy" person, or they conjure up an old Red Skelton or vaudeville routine. Yet, on the other hand, you're fully aware that there's nothing funny going on and there is nothing to laugh at.

Tourette Syndrome is characterized by sudden, repetitive, *unvoluntary* movements of one or more muscle groups, and by multiple vocalizations. The term *unvoluntary* is used rather than *involuntary* because most people with TS have a premonitory sense of the urge to tic and often can voluntarily suppress movements and vocal tics anywhere from seconds to hours. Eventually, however, the tics must be expressed, and when they are, it is often with more force and frequency.

In addition, there are numerous other symptoms that *may* be present—such as *echo phenomena* or *echolalia* (repeating the words or gestures of others), *coprolalia* (the involuntary outburst of obscene words or socially inappropriate and derogatory comments), or *palilalia* (repeating one's own words), just to mention a few—but these symptoms do *not* need to be present in order to make the TS diagnosis.

Diagnostic Criteria

Tourette Syndrome is called a *syndrome* rather than a *disease* because it presents with a number of symptoms that occur together. The diagnosis is made by taking a complete family and personal history and by observing these symptoms. At present, there is no medical test—biological or psychological—that confirms or denies the presence of Tourette Syndrome in an individual.

Because there are other conditions, including various tic disorders (such as transient childhood tics and chronic motor tics), that share some of the same symptoms, specific guidelines were compiled in the 1980s to help physicians and other professionals in making the proper diagnosis of Tourette Syndrome. These criteria are updated as more is known through research about this disorder.

According to the American Psychiatric Association's *Diagnostic and Statistical Manual of Mental Disorders* (known as *DSM-IV*), the following five symptoms *must* be present in order for a TS diagnosis to be made:

A. Both multiple motor and one or more vocal tics have been present at some time during the illness, although not necessarily concurrently. (A *tic* is a sudden, rapid, recurrent, nonrhythmic, stereotyped motor movement or vocalization.)

B. The tics occur many times a day (usually in bouts) nearly every day or intermittently throughout a period of more than one year, and during this period there was never a tic-free period of more than three consecutive months.

C. The disturbance causes marked distress or significant impairment in social, occupational, or other important areas of functioning.

D. The onset is before age eighteen years.

E. The disturbance is not due to the direct physiological effects of a substance (e.g., stimulants) or a general medical condition (e.g., Huntington's disease or postviral encephalitis.[1]

Over the last two decades, most people (including some medical professionals) first learned about Tourette Syndrome from television shows such as *Quincy, L.A. Law, Geraldo,* and others, as well as from numerous newspaper and magazine articles. Syndicated columnists such as Ann Landers have also added to the media exposure. This information explosion has had both positive and negative ramifications. While the media attention has helped immensely to educate the general public about the existence of Tourette Syndrome—and thus encouraged many families and adults to finally seek help—the popular media, unfortunately, usually tend to focus on the sensational, extreme, and bizarre aspects of TS, especially cursing.

Actually, only about 10–30 percent of those with Tourette Syndrome develop coprolalia (the medical term for this type of vocalization). Nevertheless, when friends and even some physicians heard that I was writing a book about Tourette Syndrome, many of them responded with, "Oh yes. It's that disease where people swear."

That perception is not unique. Sadly, even today many physicians still underdiagnose the disorder believing (incorrectly) that coprolalia or echolalia (involuntary repetition of another person's last word, phrase, or sentence) *must* be present for multiple vocal and motor tics to be diagnosed as TS. Despite overwhelming evidence that intellectual powers are *not* lessened by Tourette Syndrome, some doctors also look for intellectual deterioration before making a diagnosis.

Nevertheless, despite once being considered a rare disorder, new cases are being identified daily, probably because the

---

[1] Reprinted by permission of the American Psychiatric Association: *Diagnostic and Statistical Manual of Mental Disorders,* Fourth Edition (Washington, D.C.; American Psychiatric Association, 1994).

syndrome now is more commonly recognized. While there are no absolute figures of how many people in the United States have TS, most researchers agree that it is far more common than once believed. Tics of all types occur in about 35 million people in the United States alone. How many of them actually have Tourette Syndrome is difficult for investigators to evaluate for a number of reasons, including:

- People with mild TS symptoms often don't seek medical help.
- Physicians often use different (sometimes improper) criteria to make the diagnosis.
- Many cases of TS are misdiagnosed as nervous conditions, disruptive behavior, or allergies.

Some genetic studies suggest that the figure of those with the gene for Tourette Syndrome may be as high as *one in two hundred*—1.3 million people in the United States—*if* we include those with chronic multiple tics and/or transient childhood tics.

According to the Tourette Syndrome Association, "In its complete form, TS may affect up to one person in every 2,500, with perhaps three times that number showing partial expressions such as chronic tic disorder and OCD."[2]

Tourette Syndrome seems to affect people from every corner of the world. Not only have cases been reported in the United States and Europe, but also in Canada, South America, Australia, Russia, Korea, Japan, China, India, and the Middle East—people of all races, social and economic groups.

Appearance of Symptoms

The symptoms of Tourette Syndrome begin anywhere from early childhood to adolescence, usually between the ages of two and

---

[2] "Facts You Should Know About the Genetics of Tourette Syndrome" brochure, TSA, Inc.

sixteen, although some cases have emerged as late as age twenty-one. (However, some experts speculate that those symptoms actually appeared earlier, but were not recognized.) TS affects three boys for every girl. (Some studies suggest that the ratio is higher.) At present, there is no scientific explanation for this statistic, although some researchers suspect this may be due to hormonal differences between males and females as they develop.

Typically, TS symptoms begin with a simple facial tic such as a blink or twitch of the mouth or nose. Studies by Dr. Arthur Shapiro and others determined that tics around the upper part of the face—the eyes and eyelids—occurred in 80 percent of those with Tourette Syndrome. Initially, there may be sounds—a cough, grunt, or sniff.

When concerned parents take their child to the pediatrician, the ENT (ears, nose, throat) specialist (otolaryngologist), and/or the ophthalmologist, the youngster may be treated with antibiotics, allergy shots, or antihistamines. Physicians may warn the parents about too much tension in the home that is triggering this nervous habit, or they may dismiss the tic as "a simple transient childhood tic," which occurs in 15–24 percent of schoolchildren. They assure the parents that it will go away, which it will if it *is* a simple, transient childhood tic.

However, if it is Tourette Syndrome, the tic can and does become more complicated. Soon it involves more than one muscle group. The previous simple head jerk or blink may be replaced by a complex series of tics, such as lip smacking, hissing, followed by a shoulder jerk, and the child's stomach muscles tensing and tightening. Or it could become a sniff, hoot or cough, neck stretch or jerk, a hand wave followed by a foot stomping or hopping routine—or a myriad of other multiple vocal and motor tics in varying patterns, the severity of which may fluctuate from day-to-day and also with the time of day and situation.

COPROLALIA

Although often considered synonymous with Tourette Syndrome, coprolalia, the outburst of obscene or socially unacceptable words or phrases, is actually found in only 10–30 percent of those with TS (sometimes less, depending on the particular study). But for those who cannot mask the words or substitute something more socially acceptable, coprolalia is the most disturbing verbal tic.

The person with coprolalia finds himself or herself quietly walking down the street or engaging in normal conversation, then suddenly muttering or shouting out an unacceptable word or phrase, which may include ethnic or religious slurs or references to anatomy, sexual acts, bodily functions, and other derogatory words or phrases. The utterance seldom reflects the thoughts or opinions of the person saying them. As with other tics, coprolalia often is worse at home when the individual feels safer and less need to inhibit the outburst.

Coprolalia causes trouble at school, causes workers to lose their jobs, and closes many doors on social acceptance and peer support. Some who cannot control their utterances become recluses while others learn to mask their words—for example, saying "Fake" rather than the less acceptable four-letter word—mumble, or cover their mouths to muffle the words. Occasionally, those with coprolalia are able to satisfy that tic by just thinking the thoughts (known as *mental coprolalia*) rather than saying the words aloud.

Although the exact cause of this bizarre tic is unknown, researchers speculate that it is triggered by the short-circuiting of the "guard system" in our central nervous system—the one that usually inhibits us from making these utterances. Medications such as Haldol may help to suppress this tic.

COPROPRAXIA

This is a complex motor tic that incorporates involuntary obscene and otherwise socially unacceptable actions such as "giving the finger" or grabbing or pointing at one's own or someone else's breasts or genitals. While copropraxia occurs only in a small number of cases, it can be highly embarrassing and the reactions of others can be potentially dangerous to the well-being of those who cannot control this symptom.

ECHOLALIA

This vocal symptom is the involuntary repetition of another person's last word, phrase, or sentence. Occasionally, someone may repeat a sound, such as a dog barking or a cat mewing. Sometimes the repetition is done mentally so that others don't know it is occurring. Unfortunately, as the sound or words echo in the individual's head, he or she may not hear what else is being said. This distraction can have disastrous effects in school and work situations.

ECHOPRAXIA

Those with echopraxia involuntarily imitate gestures of others. This too can anger others who may believe they are being mocked or, perhaps, threatened.

PALILALIA

This is the repetition of one's own last word, phrase, or sentence.

One of the difficulties doctors have in confirming the diagnosis of Tourette Syndrome is that the type, frequency, intensity, and combination of tics are seldom the same in any two patients. In addition, many suppress their tics in the doctors' offices or similar situations, leading the doctor to doubt the descriptions of the tics.

There really is no "typical" TS case because there are so many variables not only in the type and combination of tics, but also in age of onset, fluctuation, and duration of tics as well as possible concurrent problems such as hyperactivity, attention deficits, obsessive-compulsive disorders, and self-injurious behavior.

What is typical, however, is that all of the tics are unvoluntary, sudden, rapid, and purposeless. They are repeated endlessly, sometimes to the point of actually physically exhausting the child (as well as the family, teachers, and peers who observe them).

Symptoms May Be Masked or Substituted

Recently, a great deal has been written about *premonitory* or *sensory* urges with Tourette Syndrome. Originally reported in 1980 by Joe Bliss, a man with TS, researchers began to study whether or not someone with Tourette Syndrome knew or could actually sense that a tic was about to occur. Was there, indeed, a warning signal? Until that time, tics were believed to be strictly involuntary. The results were surprising. In one seven-day study, "Ninety-three percent of 132 respondents . . . identified having a sensation (mental or physical awareness) ('an urge,' 'a feeling,' 'an impulse,' 'a need') to experience a tic."[3] Some of the patients in this study described their premonitory sensations this way:

A twenty-four-year-old man said, "A feeling of pressure—a need that's very hard to describe, like something itches deep inside you—but no place you can describe; and the only way you can relieve this need is by tics. It's like your brain itches, or your insides are being tickled."

A twenty-seven-year-old woman in that same study explained: "I guess it's sort of an aching feeling, in a limb or a body area, or else in my throat if it precedes a vocalization. If I don't relieve it, it either drives me crazy or begins to hurt (or both)—in that way it's both mental and physical."

Because of this advanced warning system, many adults and even children with TS become very adept at masking their symptoms when others are around.

When I feel my own neck tic coming on, I'll mask it by rubbing the back of my neck, especially if I think someone has spotted me jerking my head. Then I'll mumble something like, "I've got a bad stiff neck today," or I'll frown as though it's never happened before. Those who hoot, yelp, or grunt may accent the initial word of a sentence, such as "SAY THERE . . . wasn't that a great movie?" Nose twitchers or those with tongue thrusts may cover

---

[3] Leckman, James F., M.D., David E. Walker, B.A., and Donald J. Cohen, M.D., "Premonitory Urges in Tourette's Syndrome," *American Journal of Psychiatry* 150:1, January 1993.

their nose or mouth. An attorney admitted to me that he does "funny finger movements," but then he's learned to do them behind his back, under the table, or in his coat pocket. Still others take refuge by calling their tics "habits," figuring that the euphemism makes the tics seem more normal to others.

Symptoms May Be Temporarily Inhibited

Ironically, these movements and utterances can often be suppressed to some degree—as our daughter had often done with the physicians who examined her. But for the child or adult who cannot hold back, there may be embarrassment, frustration, and, without the unconditional continued support of the family, a damaged self-image. People may stare, snicker, taunt, and tease as they often do when faced with anyone who is "different." A movie, ballet, concert, or church service becomes a lengthy anxiety-filled attempt to avoid disturbing others. What's more, the stress and fatigue from the great effort that suppressing entails often serves only to make the tics far worse than usual.

"You become entangled in a delicate balance," a father of a ten-year-old with Tourette Syndrome told me. "As a parent, you believe wholeheartedly that your child has the same rights as everyone else. For example, she should be able to attend a Broadway show like any other kid with chronic disabilities. But then you start thinking, what about the rights of the others who also have paid good money to see that hit musical? Surely they have some right to enjoy the show. If your child is yelping or jumping around in her seat—even if she can't help it—it disturbs others and they can't have a good time. I feel torn. My wife and I fight about this all the time. She says I'm being disloyal to our daughter, but I'm just trying to figure out what's fair. It's not a black-or-white issue. There's mostly gray areas."

TS Symptoms Wax and Wane

Another source of tension for a family is the tendency of TS tics to wax and wane throughout one's lifetime. Just when everyone involved thinks they cannot stand to hear (or do) one more throat clearing, sniff, or grunt, or to watch (or perform) a specific combination of motor tics that often becomes physically painful to overworked muscles and joints, the tics "magically" disappear for a few days, weeks, or even months.

The first time this happens, the thought hovers in everyone's mind that perhaps the doctors were mistaken. Perhaps it isn't Tourette Syndrome at all, just transient tics. Even after the family becomes used to the waxing and waning phenomenon, it's still easy to get caught up in that hope. As soon as it registers that "Hey, Tommy isn't doing those tics anymore," everyone breathes a sigh of relief, even though they know better. Maybe *this* time they won't return. Typically, the tics do return, if not in the same form, then in another.

"When the new tic is worse than the old," one mother admitted, "it makes you wish the familiar nose twitch were back."

This fluctuating pattern, the "now you see it, now you don't," occurrence is described by many as one of the more difficult parts of coping with TS. "I can deal with my son's tics," more than one parent confessed, "but I feel like Charlie Brown every time the tics go away and I think, I pray . . . maybe *this* time . . . Then, like Lucy with the football, that hope gets pulled away. It's cruel."

"Parents of kids with TS go through phases," said Dr. Roger Freeman, a child psychiatrist and director of the Neuropsychiatry Clinic of Children's Hospital in Vancouver, British Columbia. "At first they're anxious when their child develops a new tic. But after this cycle has been repeated many times, they get used to it.

"Parents also worry that the tic is causing their child pain," he continued. "That's a source of confusion. Often it really isn't pain, but rather an inner discomfort sensation.

"There seems to be a high rate of knuckle cracking . . . in a set sequence. First they crack their neck, then their back, then sometimes on down to the toes. My patients tell me they have to keep doing it until 'it feels right.' It's like there's an endless loop and some subsystem doesn't shut off."

Many individuals with TS echoed this "has to feel right"

phrase. "I have to jerk my neck until I feel a 'click,' " a young man told me. Another said he repeated a low barking noise until "it's right." No one was able to put into words just what made a tic feel "right," or describe a "right" feeling.

One teenager's tic repertoire included smashing her hand against a concrete wall. When her mother suggested that she might consider wearing gloves to protect her hand, the youngster replied, "But then it wouldn't have the same sensation; it wouldn't 'feel right.' "

Tactile Sensitivity

Any writer (or researcher, for that matter) unconsciously somewhat skews a study because he or she asks certain questions and omits others. Obviously, interviewees might offer additional comments if asked about a particular issue, but otherwise might not mention anything, considering it to be unimportant.

Two of my children with TS had complained of skin sensitivities—one used to wear pajamas under his dress pants because otherwise they felt "itchy." (To this day he won't wear woolen sweaters.) I wondered if others with TS had the same tactile sensitivity too. So I included that question in most of my professional and lay interviews.

To my surprise, many respondents said they had never mentioned it before because no one had ever asked. When comparing notes with many TS professionals, I quickly learned that this phenomenon is called *sensory integrative disorder* and is not uncommon. It's found among those *without* TS as well. It's like a hypersensitivity of the senses.

One man with a mild case of TS said he too had worn long-legged pajamas under his wool suit pants as a youngster. "My Bar Mitzvah picture shows a bit of the p.j.'s hanging down from my trousers," he laughed.

Others mentioned an inability to wear turtleneck shirts. "They make my neck tic worse," two women said. Children described feeling uncomfortable walking barefoot in the sand or on grass, and not wanting to play with clay or other "gooey" substances.

Both children and adults complained about "scratchy" labels in shirts, tight clothing that irritated, and new clothing not feeling "right." Dr. Freeman said many of his TS patients don't wear socks because the seams don't feel "right."

This information is important because many of the resulting behaviors caused by this tactile insensitivity can be misperceived as a behavioral problem. Teachers may interpret a child's refusal to fingerpaint or paste cutouts as being oppositional behavior, because they don't understand that the feel of the paint or paste actually bothers the youngster. Similarly, if Mom understands why her daughter refuses to wear socks, prefers old or baggy clothes, and won't wear wool, or gags on lumps in mashed potatoes or food with raisins in it, she may not take it personally, so power struggles can be avoided.

Some of those with TS also indicated an auditory sensitivity, finding sirens or loud music truly painful to their ears. Numerous adults, including myself, find it difficult to concentrate with music or other sound in the background. I have always admired those who can write in a newspaper or TV news room.

It isn't yet clear from comparative research whether these observations are really more common in TS than in other neuropsychiatric disorders. Perhaps ongoing research may help to resolve this.

Future Outlook for Someone with TS

Despite the frustrating features of Tourette Syndrome, there are positive aspects to consider. Although there is no cure for TS, it is *not* a life-threatening disease, nor does it shorten life expectancy.

Tourette Syndrome tics usually tend to disappear when a person is totally focused, such as playing the piano or video games, working on a computer, or meditating.

In addition, for some youngsters with TS, the symptoms seem to lessen to some degree upon reaching late adolescence. Most people with Tourette Syndrome do lead normal and productive lives. According to researchers Harvey S. Singer, M.D., and

John T. Walkup, M.D., "It has been estimated that in 30–40 percent of children with TS all tic symptoms will disappear by late adolescence, and in an additional 30 percent, tics will diminish markedly." They add, however, that the remaining patients will have some symptoms—usually not worse than in childhood—persisting into their adult years.

For those individuals with mild symptoms, few of their coworkers or friends will take any notice of their tics. Of course, family members will be aware, because most people with Tourette Syndrome tend to relax at home, knowing they are "safe" in giving their tics full expression. A father who had a barking tic voiced only at home overheard his daughter on the telephone saying matter-of-factly to a friend, "Oh, we don't have a dog. That's my father."

For those whose tics are more severe, life in the adult world is somewhat more difficult. Sometimes deprived of self-confidence by TS in their adolescent years, they enter adulthood ill-prepared for social and business relationships.

Perhaps, one day soon, the cure will be found to make the tics of Tourette Syndrome disappear forever, but even if that were to happen, many of these adults still would lack some of the skills most learn during childhood and adolescence. How to make up for lost years is a problem yet to be resolved.

CHAPTER 4

Exposing the Myths

When you first are diagnosed with any disease or disorder, new, confusing, and conflicting information can quickly create an emotional overload, adding to your already present burden of anxiety and stress. That's why it is important to understand what Tourette Syndrome is, in order to help your child, yourself, your family, and those with whom you are in contact. Because TS is such an unusual and greatly misunderstood disorder, a great many myths have traveled with it throughout the years, confusing those who sincerely want to be supportive, delaying diagnosis, and creating an even greater trauma for those who must find ways to adapt to living with it.

Myth #1: *People with Tourette Syndrome are suffering from a mental disorder.* False. Although emotional problems may arise from trying to cope with the effects of TS symptoms, Tourette Syndrome is a biological disorder of the central nervous system. While OCD and ADD with or without hyperactivity may be additional components of the disorder, the majority of those with TS don't experience these conditions.

Myth #2: *There has to be coprolalia (i.e., swearing and "dirty" words) in order for a condition to be diagnosed as Tourette Syndrome.* False. Coprolalia is *not* one of the American Psychiatric Association's criteria needed in order to make the diagnosis of TS. In fact, experts report that far less than 30 percent of those with Tourette Syndrome have coprolalia as one of their symptoms. The majority of these people can mask the words, by saying, "F . . . FINE," rather than the offending four-letter word.

Unfortunately, because this symptom is a "sensational" one, it seems to be the one referred to most frequently on television shows and in newspaper and magazine articles about TS. While it's good to have the general public informed about Tourette Syndrome, it isn't helpful to keep perpetuating the myth that coprolalia is a typical symptom of TS. It isn't.

Myth #3: *A person with TS tics could stop them if he or she really wanted to.* False. This myth may be perpetuated by the fact that tics *can* be inhibited for a short time. Then, however, as explained previously, the pressure builds up and the person can no longer hold them back; they must be expressed, sometimes more forcefully than before.

Myth #4: *Hypnosis is effective in controlling the tics.* False. Although it seems as though *everything* is effective at first due to the waxing and waning phenomenon of Tourette Syndrome tics, hypnosis is not a means of controlling tics. It can, however, be used to promote relaxation and the reduction of stress, which in turn may help to reduce the intensity and frequency of the tics.

Myth #5: *Tourette Syndrome causes intellectual deterioration.* False. There is no study demonstrating that TS causes deterioration of intellectual powers. Even Gilles de la Tourette stressed that point in his original paper in 1885. However, children often have difficulty in an academic setting because of their tics, which may interfere with their ability to read, write, concentrate, or follow instructions.

In addition, the OCD and/or ADD with or without hyperactivity components that may co-occur can create a greater burden in the learning process. Side effects from medication given to reduce tics also can play a part in learning difficulties.

Myth #6: *Someone with Tourette Syndrome will never be able to have a "normal" life.* False. While TS is a chronic or remitting disorder, the tics tend to disappear or become less noticeable as a person enters adulthood in the majority of cases. With some exceptions, most adults who want or need to work find jobs and/or rewarding careers.

Myth #7: *A person will stop ticcing if you bring the tic to his or her attention every time he or she does it.* False. People with Tourette Syndrome usually know when they are ticcing. You certainly don't need to point it out. In fact, focusing on the tics may actually increase stress, thus escalating the tics' frequency and/or intensity. Even if they are not aware of their tics, your pointing them out cannot help them to stop.

Myth #8: *Tourette Syndrome is caused by faulty parenting techniques.* False. Although poor parenting skills can create additional stress within a family, it does *not* cause Tourette Syndrome. As stated before, TS is caused by a chemical imbalance in the brain. It is a neurobiological disorder, not a psychogenic one.

Myth #9: *All children with Tourette Syndrome will outgrow it once they reach adulthood.* False. While many people with TS have a lessening of symptoms, and some may experience a total remission in their late teens, others carry it with them throughout adulthood.

Myth #10: *If you have Tourette Syndrome, your tics will prevent you from playing sports.* False. There are a number of outstanding professional athletes with Tourette Syndrome. Two of the best known are Jim Eisenreich and Mahmoud Abdul-Rauf, whose success stories are found in Chapter 24.

Myth #11: *People with Tourette Syndrome are possessed by the devil and need to be cured by exorcism.* False. While history suggests that some "witches" burned at the stake may have been people suffering from Tourette Syndrome, people with this disorder are not possessed by the devil. Instead, they suffer from a chemical imbalance in the brain. According to Drs. Arthur and Elaine Shapiro and others, "A rejuvenated interest in exorcism has been stimulated by the movie *The Exorcist,* which is reputedly based on an exaggerated and distorted interpretation of a patient with Tourette Syndrome who had been hospitalized at Georgetown University.''[1]

Myth #12: *Giving children medication for their tics will make them more likely to become involved in street drugs.* False. There are no studies to show that children with Tourette Syndrome who use medication to control their tics are more likely to be involved with drug abuse.

Myth #13: *All doctors are well informed about Tourette Syndrome and know how best to treat it.* False. Unfortunately, even today many physicians and other health-care professionals know little, if anything, about TS. Some of them actually help to perpetuate some of the myths concerning TS or are relying on outdated material to advise them. In addition, as you probably have already discovered, there are many areas of disagreement even among those most informed about this disorder. Some researchers, for example, feel strongly that ADHD and/or OCD are a part of the possible expression of TS, whereas others are just as insistent that they are separate disorders having no connection. You as the parent or patient may feel frustrated as you try to sort out the divergent thinking. ''Why can't all these doctors agree?'' one parent asked.

The answer? ''They seldom do at this stage of our knowledge.''

Myth #14: *Having Tourette Syndrome shortens a person's life expectancy.* False. Although Tourette Syndrome is a chronic disorder, it is *not* life threatening, nor does it shorten one's life expectancy. The reason you may not hear of too many elderly people with Tourette Syndrome is that it wasn't diagnosed when they were children and their tics may have lessened as they

---

[1] Shapiro, Arthur K., Elaine S. Shapiro, Ruth D. Bruun, and Richard D. Sweet, *Gilles de la Tourette Syndrome* (New York: Raven, 1978).

became older. These people also have had many years to become used to their symptoms and probably consider them just part of what is their "normal" behavior. It's unlikely that they would seek medical care for these lifelong tics.

Obviously, people who have Tourette Syndrome *do* die, but it isn't from having TS.

Myth #15: *All people with TS express the same symptoms.* False. While there are similarities in the tics themselves, the combinations, severity, and frequency differ from person to person.

Myth #16: *TS occurs only in certain ethnic groups.* False. TS has been found in all ethnic groups.

Myth #17: *TS can be diagnosed by a medical test.* False. To date there is no medical test that can be given to determine whether or not an individual has TS. Diagnosis must be made by observation of the symptoms (which often are suppressed in the doctor's office) and by taking a complete medical history.

Myth #18: *A person cannot be hurt by his or her motor tics.* False. Some motor tics can cause injury. Over time, severe neck jerking has been known to trigger muscle pain and neck spasms, herniate cervical disks, and in extremely rare cases, rupture the vertebral or carotid arteries that carry blood to the brain, resulting in a stroke, or injury to the spinal cord, causing quadriplegia.

Arm or leg jerking tics can injure muscles over time as well. In addition, some individuals with Tourette Syndrome suffer from self-injurious behavior (SIB). It can range from hitting oneself (and others) to lip biting, picking at nails until they bleed, and head-banging.

Myth #19: *There is little that patients or their families can do to help researchers learn more about TS.* False. In addition to donating funds to help researchers, families with TS can volunteer to participate in research studies. In addition, the TSA Brain Bank program urges those with TS to sign up to donate their brain at the time of their death. Almost no autopsy information has ever been obtained on people with TS because there is no tissue to study. This means that scientists have never systematically studied the brain mechanisms of those with Tourette Syndrome.

No chronic illness occurs in a vacuum. It has rippling effects on all who come in contact, changing everyone. These adaptations, however, need not be negative. Many people acknowledge that having to deal with Tourette Syndrome has made themselves, family members, and friends more caring and understanding of the problems of others.

Yes, TS *is* a chronic disorder, but it is not a life-threatening one. While there are numerous difficulties that must be acknowledged and faced, please take comfort in the knowledge that most families do work out satisfactory coping techniques, so that although Tourette Syndrome is part of their lives, it does not become their entire lives.

CHAPTER 5

Understanding the Cause
and Treatment

One of the most common questions asked about Tourette Syndrome is, "How do you get it?" Often there's an unspoken concern that perhaps TS is contagious and can be "caught" like mumps or the chicken pox.

Tourette Syndrome often appears within the same family; it's not uncommon to see a parent and child, or two or more siblings, with TS. That's because there's a genetic tendency to having Tourette Syndrome, not because it is catching.

Although researchers have not, as yet, been able to identify a genetic marker for TS, "late 20th-century neurological views implicate hypersensitivity of dopamine receptors in the substantia nigra [a midbrain structure] pathway as the possible underlying neurological factor in TS behaviors."[1]

Dopamine, one of many chemicals found in the brain, is a neurotransmitter, a substance that controls movement by sending messages across gaps between nerve cells called synapses. There may be additional neurotransmitters involved in causing TS as well, including one called *serotonin.*

Present studies suggest that Tourette Syndrome is genetically

---

[1] Kushner, Howard I., Ph.D., and Louise S. Kiessling, M.D., FAAP, "Rethinking the Diagnostic Boundaries of TS: The Possible Role of Strepto-coccal Antibodies in TS," Tourette Syndrome Association, Inc. Newsletter, Vol. XXI, No. 4, 1993–94. Reprinted by permission.

transmitted in most instances, although some cases have been thought to be triggered by trauma to the brain.

Georges Gilles de la Tourette suggested that there might be a genetic basis for the disorder when he first studied his group of nine afflicted patients back in 1885. Nevertheless, there was little follow-up research on his findings until almost a century later. The prevailing theory held by physicians until well into the late 1960s and early 1970s was that TS had a *psychological* basis.

Hundreds of frantic parents were singled out for poor parenting techniques, which led, so it was said, to their child's "acting out of frustrations or trying for attention through verbal and motor tics." Parents ran from doctor to doctor for help, some seeing as many as ten to thirty physicians before finally receiving a proper diagnosis.

Finally, in the mid-1960s, Drs. Arthur and Elaine Shapiro, Ruth D. Bruun, Richard D. Sweet, and others began to examine their ever-growing patient base, searching for scientific data to support their belief that Tourette Syndrome had a biological and not a psychological cause. Then and until quite recently, many obstacles existed. Researchers disagreed on diagnostic criteria. Was obsessive-compulsive disorder a part of TS or merely a closely related disorder? What about attention deficit disorder? Hyperactivity? Were chronic tics a form of TS or the manifestation of another disorder altogether? Was TS a spectrum disorder, and if so, why was it mild in some and severe in others? If the disorder were genetic, exactly how was it passed from one generation to another?

These are not simple questions or unimportant ones. Without a common standard of evaluation, no one can be certain that the growing number of independent researchers were investigating the same issues with similar cases. In science, facts must be replicated in order to be considered proven. There needs to be a sufficient number of patients that can be compared with a control group of people without TS symptoms. Lastly, and probably most important of all in those early days, there needed to be continual communication among these researchers, most of whom were grossly underfunded because Tourette Syndrome was then considered to be such a rare disorder.

To resolve these issues, finally, in 1983 the Tourette Syndrome

Association began promoting investigator-initiated research. Three years later, they expanded their Scientific Advisory Board, adding a Subcommittee for Genetics. Today, supported by the Tourette Syndrome Association grant awards, scientists throughout North America and Europe collaborate in an exciting effort to map the elusive gene or genes responsible for Tourette Syndrome. At this writing—and I intentionally use this qualifier because success in genetic sleuthing occurs daily and often because of unexpected breakthroughs—the specific gene(s) responsible for Tourette Syndrome has not been located.

According to researchers Ben J. M. van de Wetering and P. Heutink of the Netherlands, "Once a convincing linkage has been found, the job of cloning the GTS gene(s) will start. With the gene(s) in hand, the study of the interaction between the inherited vulnerability and environmental factors in the pathogenesis (i.e., the origins of the development of a disease) will come to its ultimate challenge. These insights will provide the future key to a more rational treatment and optimal support for the patient with GTS and his relatives who are at risk.[2]

According to the Tourette Syndrome Association,[3] the genetic vulnerability to TS is transmitted from one (or both) gene-carrying parent to the male or female offspring. The precise expression and severity may differ from one generation to another. That means if one parent has TS or is a TS gene carrier, there is about a 50 percent chance that each child born to that couple may inherit the genetic vulnerability for a tic spectrum disorder. (This mode of inheritance is called *autosomal dominant.*)

But it's important to remember that not every child who inherits the genetic vulnerability for TS will display symptoms. Some may be silent carriers. (When a gene does not always cause symptoms, it is called *incomplete penetrance.*) Often the degree of penetrance (expression of symptoms) is different in males and females.

With Tourette Syndrome, there is about a 70 percent chance

---

[2] van de Wetering, Ben J. M., and P. Heutink, "The Genetics of the Gilles de la Tourette Syndrome: A Review," Mosby Year Book, Inc., 1993.
[3] Adapted by permission of the Tourette Syndrome Association from their booklet, "The Genetics of Tourette Syndrome."

that a female child *who has inherited the genetic tendency* will have some symptoms of TS. A male child *who has inherited the gene* is believed to have about a 99 percent chance of showing some symptoms of TS sometime in his life. (Some studies, however, show lower percentages.) Thus, the expression of symptoms is sex-specific for Tourette Syndrome, with the male-female ratio being 4:1 or even 3:1, depending on which research data are used. There is a full 30 percent chance that female gene carriers will show no symptoms at all, with only a one percent chance for males.

The gene (or genes) for TS creates different symptoms in different people. There is a range of forms the symptoms may take, including full-blown "textbook" TS, chronic tic disorder, OCD, and possibly, transient tic disorder or ADHD, although there is disagreement by experts on the latter. Some individuals may have TS and OC symptoms, whereas others may have just one condition. Males are more likely to have TS or chronic tics, whereas females are more likely to have OC symptoms. However, both male and female offspring may express any combination of symptoms or any degree of severity.

In addition, it is wishful thinking to assume that a child's tics won't be as severe as the parents because there's no guarantee. No one can predict the severity of symptoms based on those of the parent. Do remember, however, that *most individuals who inherit the TS genetic vulnerability have very mild conditions for which they do not seek medical attention.*

Actually, according to many studies, only about 10 percent of children who do inherit the TS gene will ever experience symptoms severe enough to require medical attention. Most people with TS have such mild symptoms that they never become patients and are never diagnosed by health-care professionals. That's one of the reasons that it's difficult to determine how many people actually have TS.

Dr. Freeman stressed that, "You have to distinguish between the community population as a whole and the children we see in the clinic. We tend to see those children with moderate to severe symptoms, as well as those for whom the symptoms, however mild they may be, are troublesome to either the child or to the parents. They also may have other behaviors that are creating problems. I believe the majority of TS cases cause so little difficulty that they remain medically undiagnosed.''

What About Genetic Counseling?

Although knowledgeable physicians and/or genetic counselors can tell a couple what is known about the genetics of TS in order to help them make family planning decisions, at present there are no genetic or biochemical tests available to determine whether or not a person is a carrier for Tourette Syndrome, or whether or not a child might develop the condition. Also, if the baby were to inherit TS, there is no prenatal test to determine the type of symptoms or their severity. The development of these various diagnostic tests must wait in the shadows until the TS gene is discovered.

That's why researchers have combined their efforts in an encouraging display of scientific cooperation. Locating a genetic marker for TS would provide a way to determine which individuals are carriers. The next challenge is to locate the abnormal gene itself, determine what went wrong, and work toward developing medications specifically for Tourette Syndrome. As Sue Levi-Pearl, medical liaison for the TSA stated, ''All the medications now used to treat TS were created to help other types of medical conditions. We need something specifically designed for TS and, ideally, a medicine without side effects.''

The last and final goal for TS researchers, of course, is to discover a cure for this disorder. May that time not be far off.

Possible Additional Causes

In the early 1990s, research at the National Institute of Mental Health (NIMH) and Memorial Hospital of Rhode Island (MHRI) suggested that antibodies to strep infection may provide the environmental trigger in genetically susceptible families for a variety of movement disorders *including* Tourette Syndrome.

Investigators[4] "speculate that an immunologic reaction to neuronal [nerve cell] tissue set off by these streptococcal products contributes to the development of tics . . . and their combinations as well as to obsessive compulsive symptoms."

This research may demonstrate that there is a family history of tics, OCD, or ADHD, including those associated with rheumatic fever. Until it is definitive, however, the researchers recommend that, "For new onset tic disorders or acute relapses . . . the family's physician tests for evidence of streptococcal infection. If such an infection is diagnosed, it should be treated vigorously with antibiotics. At this point, however, **there is no confirmed commonly available selective intervention for tic symptoms that have arisen as a result of the presence of these antibodies.** There are, however, several pilot studies underway at NIMH under the direction of Dr. Susan Swedo, Director of Behavioral Pediatrics at NIMH's child psychiatry section. The hope is that ongoing research will lead to appropriate and effective treatments."[5]

As far as we presently know, environmental factors *of themselves* do not cause TS. However, there is little doubt that stress and tension may adversely affect the frequency and intensity of the tics.

Many of the TS symptoms, such as sniffing, throat clearing, nose twitching, blinking, lip licking, and coughing can mimic those of allergies. Pediatricians, allergists, and otolaryngologists who see children with these symptoms should remain alert for other motor and vocal tics and consider the possible diagnosis of TS in these patients. While most TS experts believe that allergy is not related to Tourette Syndrome in any way, there is an alternative school of thought that suggests that treatment of

---

[4] Swedo, Susan, M.D., H. L. Leonard, M. B. Schapiro, Louise S. Kiessling, M.D., FAAP, A. C. Marcotte, L. Culpepper, J. L. Rapoport, B. S. Cheslow, and others.

[5] Kushner, Howard I., Ph.D., and Louise S. Kiessling, M.D., FAAP, "Rethinking the Diagnostic Boundaries of TS: The Possible Role of Streptococcal Antibodies in TS," Tourette Syndrome Association, Inc. Newsletter, Vol. XXI, No. 4, 1993–94. Reprinted by permission.

allergies may help to relieve some of the symptoms of TS. It's also important to remember that children with Tourette Syndrome are first and foremost children, and may have many of the same problems that kids without TS have. They can have allergies, just as they also can be myopic and/or have asthma.

Treatment

It's fairly typical that shortly after most people hear the diagnosis of Tourette Syndrome, the first question is, "Is there a cure?" Unfortunately, as of this writing, the answer must be "no." However, because of the waxing and waning phenomenon of the symptoms, almost everything at one time or another—from antidepressants and acupuncture to hypnosis, lobotomy, and shock therapy—has been touted as being the "cure."

In the early seventies, Drs. Arthur and Elaine Shapiro said, "Everything works with Tourette Syndrome . . . for a while." What they meant was that because of the tendency of TS tics to wax and wane, you often feel as though you've hit on the exact treatment, only to discover that it was tried during the waning phase of the tics and they would have improved anyway.

The good news, however, is that there are many different treatments—both medical and nonmedical—that have proven effective in reducing the severity and frequency of the tics in some people some of the time. Nothing works for everyone all of the time. The uniqueness of each person's symptoms makes it impossible to treat TS—and many other disorders—in a rigid "one size fits all" manner.

There is a vast difference in the types, severity, and frequency of symptoms expressed, ranging from extremely mild at one end to those for whom TS is a major disabling chronic illness at the other. Fortunately, the majority—70 percent or more—of those with Tourette Syndrome have mild tics and do not require any type of treatment, medical or otherwise, to help them to either control or deal with their symptoms. For these people, TS is a minor inconvenience, an occasional source of embarrassment, nothing more.

Numerous health-care professionals have mentioned seeing a youngster with TS for the first time and asking the parent (who is blinking or jerking) what other family members have tics. The parent answers, "None that I know of." It isn't that the parent is lying or is in denial. It's just that he or she really is not aware of the tics.

For those whose tics and associated behavioral problems are more troublesome, however, there is a variety of available medications that have proven helpful for many. They do not, however, totally eradicate the difficulties, and they are not effective for everyone. What's more, each medication comes with its own list of troubling side effects. Many times, individuals decide that the cure is worse than the tics and they stop treatment. Psychological support also is beneficial to bolster self-esteem and to assist with relationship problems, but neither medication nor counseling provides a cure.

In Dr. Oliver Sacks' extraordinary book, *The Man Who Mistook His Wife for a Hat,* he describes Ray, a young drummer with TS who, on medication, found himself "musically 'dull,' average, competent, but lacking energy, enthusiasm, extravagance and joy. He no longer had his tics or compulsive hitting of the drums—but he no longer had wild and creative surges."[6]

Once it has been determined to use any type of medication treatment, the goal must be to carefully *titrate* the dosage. This means using the smallest possible amount in order to minimize side effects while effecting some benefit in reducing (not totally eliminating) the most troublesome symptoms. It's a difficult balancing act because everyone reacts differently to a particular medication as well as to a specific dosage, and also these responses may vary from day to day. Children use the same medications as adults, but in smaller doses.

In addition, results usually are far from immediate, which

---

[6] Sacks goes on to say that eventually Ray made the compromise to take medication only during the workweek, and to go without it on the weekend, allowing himself to be "witty ticcy Ray," whatever he and his TS permitted him to be.

means the physician and family must often wait weeks or even months in order to find out whether a particular medication and/or dosage is the "right" one. This is frustrating and difficult. Parents must guard against trying to persuade the physician to raise the dosage in order to make "all the tics go away," as this can mean overmedicating the youngster and unnecessarily increasing side effects. Parents must honestly determine whether they want their child's medication increased because the tics are bothering the child or because they themselves find them troubling and embarrassing.

Some individuals with TS may require different medication to help with behavioral problems. This creates additional concerns. Not only must both medications individually be balanced to minimize troubling side effects while controlling tics and/or behavioral difficulties, but they also must be monitored for their combined effects. It takes a medical professional well versed in pharmacology to titrate these dosages properly.

As the medical treatment of TS is largely one of trial and error, parents and patients must work closely with their physician, understanding that the doctor is as anxious as the family to find something that works. Parents should keep carefully written notes of changes in tics or behavioral problems as well as *specific* side effects observed at each dosage increase or decrease.

Dr. Gerald Erenberg of the Cleveland Clinic Foundation and chairman of the Tourette Syndrome Association's Medical Advisory Board states in his booklet, "A Consumer's Guide to Tourette Syndrome Medications,"[7] "The neuroleptic medications (e.g., Haldol and Orap) may have an additional possible side effect known as tardive dyskinesia (TD). Symptoms are restless arm, hand, and foot movements or chewing or blowing movements which occur only rarely in persons with Tourette Syndrome, but are a potential long-term side effect which may not disappear if the medication is discontinued.

"Some of the possible side effects with neuroleptic medication can be controlled by an additional group of drugs known as

---

[7] Available through the National TSA office.

anticholinergic medications. Examples would be Artane and Cogentin. There is no need for these medications to be given routinely, but some individuals may experience a decrease in certain side effects when these medications are added to the neuroleptics."[8]

Pharmacotherapy for TS Tics

I have intentionally omitted the listing of "usual" dosages of these medications. The particular starting or maintenance dosage must be determined on an individual basis, with the family working closely with the physician to balance effectiveness of medication with side effects. Do *not* compare what your child is getting with the dosage of another youngster. There may be additional underlying factors determining this equation. Remember that no patient gets *all* side effects listed for a particular medication. Some get many; many get a few; and some get none. Also, side effects may lessen as the body becomes used to the chemical.

HALOPERIDOL (BRAND NAME: HALDOL)

First used to treat TS in 1961 and considered the "drug of choice" since the early 1970s, Haldol is one of the main medications used to treat TS.

Unfortunately, the side effects may be numerous and, in about 25 percent of the cases where it is used, debilitating. These side effects may include fatigue, weight gain, muscle rigidity, personality changes, school phobia, skin sensitivity to light, depression, and even (although rarely) tardive dyskinesia, a condition that includes involuntary chewing-like movements and tongue thrusts. While as many as 70 percent of those on Haldol find it

---

[8] Reprinted from "A Consumer's Guide to Tourette Syndrome Medications" by Gerald Erenberg, M.D., by permission of the Tourette Syndrome Association, Inc.

beneficial in reducing the frequency and severity of the tics, others, like Dr. Oliver Sacks' "Witty Ticcy Ray," often find the side effects more difficult to tolerate than having the tics.

CLONIDINE (BRAND NAME: CATAPRES)

First used to treat TS in 1979, clonidine is preferred by many physicians as the drug of choice, believing that it has fewer side effects than Haldol. According to a report by Drs. Donald J. Cohen, Mark A. Riddle, and James F. Leckman, "clonidine tends to have a slower onset of action [than Haldol]. . . . Even before tics are reduced, the patient may experience a reduction in tension, a feeling of being calm, or a sense of having a 'longer fuse.' . . . The major side effect of clonidine is sedation. . . . Irritability is the next most common side effect."[9] Additional side effects from this medication include dry mouth, dizziness, headache, and insomnia. Clonidine is also available as a skin patch, which delivers the medication at a constant rate, although it may irritate some people's skin.

PIMOZIDE (BRAND NAME: ORAP)

This medication has been used in the United States since 1984 to treat TS (much earlier in Canada). Like Haldol, it may have side effects including fatigue, weight gain, muscle rigidity, personality changes, tardive dyskinesia, school phobia, skin sensitivity to light, depression, as well as EKG (electrocardiogram) changes.

FLUPHENAZINE (BRAND NAME: PROLIXIN)

Side effects for this drug may include fatigue, weight gain, muscle rigidity, personality changes, school phobia, skin sensitivity to light, depression, and possible tardive dyskinesia.

---

[9] Cohen, Donald J., M.D., Mark A. Riddle, M.D., and James F. Leckman, M.D., "Pharmacotherapy of Tourette's Syndrome and Associated Disorders," *Psychiatric Clinics of North America*, Vol. 15, No. 1, March 1992.

CLONAZEPAM (BRAND NAME: KLONOPIN)

Side effects noticed from those taking this medication include fatigue, irritability, and dizziness.

RISPERIDONE (BRAND NAME: RISPERDAL)

This drug is fairly new and is sometimes used for poor responders to the other medications. Its possible side effects include tardive dyskinesia, irregular pulse, dizziness, impaired judgment, thinking, or motor skills.

NICOTINE PATCH

At this writing, double-blind controlled studies are being conducted to determine the long-term therapeutic benefits on the frequency and severity of TS tics of a nicotine skin patch. Earlier open trials by Drs. A. A. Silver and Paul R. Sanberg of the University of South Florida College of Medicine as well as other researchers have been promising.

Medications Used for Conditions That May Be Associated with TS

IMIPRAMINE (BRAND NAME: TOFRANIL)

One of the tricyclic antidepressants, this medicine is used to reduce the depression that sometimes accompanies TS. Its possible side effects include dry mouth, blurred vision, constipation, fatigue, EKG changes, skin sensitivity to light, and weight gain. It also is used sometimes to treat ADD and ADHD.

DESIPRAMINE (BRAND NAME: NORPRAMIN)

Used for the same purposes as imipramine, the possible side effects are similar.

NORTRIPTYLINE (BRAND NAME: PAMELOR)

Also used for accompanying depression as well as to treat ADD and ADHD, the possible side effects are the same as those of imipramine.

FLUOXETINE (BRAND NAME: PROZAC)

This drug is used as an antidepressant and is effective in reducing the severity of OCD. It also is used sometimes to treat ADD and ADHD. Possible side effects include agitation, insomnia, stomach upset or nausea, and impotency or other changes in sexual response in either sex. This problem may not be discussed with a patient when the drug is first prescribed, so the user should ask questions. Fluoxetine may suppress appetite for some individuals and is the longest lasting of this class of drugs.

PAROXETINE (PAXIL)

Paroxetine is one of the newer medications used for both OCD and depression. Its possible side effects are the same as those for fluoxetine.

FLUVOXAMINE (LUVOX)

Another medication just recently approved for use in treating depression and OCD, it also has possible side effects similar to those of fluoxetine.

CLOMIPRAMINE (ANAFRANIL)

Also used for both depression and OCD as well as for ADD and ADHD when Ritalin cannot be used, the possible side effects include dry mouth, blurred vision, constipation, dizziness, fatigue, EKG changes, sexual dysfunction, and skin sensitivity to light.

SERTRALINE (BRAND NAME: ZOLOFT)

This is used for both depression and OCD and has the same possible side effects as fluoxetine.

METHYLPHENIDATE (BRAND NAME: RITALIN)

One of the best-known medications for overactivity, distractibility, and short attention span, Ritalin helps both adults and children with ADHD and ADD to focus. Its possible side effects include headache, stomachache, appetite loss, insomnia, irritability, and in some cases, increased tics. When the problems associated with ADHD create more dysfunction than the symptoms of TS, some choose to continue to take this medication, but it should be closely monitored by a physician.

PEMOLINE (BRAND NAME: CYLERT)

Another attention stimulant medication, it has the same possible side effects as methylphenidate.

DEXTROAMPHETAMINE (BRAND NAME: DEXEDRINE)

This is another possible choice for attention stimulant medications and also has the same list of possible side effects as methylphenidate.

Should Stimulant Medications Be Used with a History of TS?

Pediatric psychiatrist Roger D. Freeman, a member of the TSA Medical Advisory Board, offered this advice to parents and physicians who are concerned about the use of stimulant drugs in attention deficit hyperactivity disorder combined with tics or Tourette Syndrome: "If you have been confused about the use of drugs commonly called 'stimulants' (Ritalin, Dexedrine, and Cylert) for Attention Deficit/Hyperactivity Disorder (AD/HD) in children with TS, it's not surprising. For some children or adolescents with both diagnoses, the AD/HD may be a more significant problem than the tics or TS. *In this brief discussion, I am assuming that a competent diagnosis of both conditions has already been made.*

"Several years ago there appeared to be some evidence that these drugs might cause—or aggravate—tics or TS. Physicians were advised not to prescribe them if there was a history of tics in the child, or even in other close members of the child's family. One of the problems in doing research on this issue is that the average age of onset of tics is around age seven, but for AD/HD it is closer to two or three years. This means that many children with AD/HD who are destined to develop tics or TS will already be on stimulant drug therapy at the time their tics start.

"Because of the time required before professionals, parents and the public become aware of new information, many people do not know that the pendulum has started to swing back in the other direction. There is much more clinical experience on which to base tentative conclusions, as well as some additional research.

"At present [Author's note: 1995] the opinion of many experts in this field is that if the AD/HD is an important problem to target, the stimulant drugs need not be withheld in patients with tics or Tourette Syndrome, even if there is a risk (in a minority of cases) that the tics might become worse. There seems little—if any—indication that such worsening is permanent." [NOTE: There are, however, mixed opinions on this matter.]

"If the tics *do* become significantly worse, then a clinical choice will have to be made to (a) tolerate the tics (as the lesser problem); (b) suppress the tics with an anti-tic medication; or (c) try a different class of drug for the AD/HD (some of which also increase tics occasionally).

"It is likely that more information will soon be available from present research studies. The Tourette Syndrome Association intends to publish additional detailed material on the treatment of AD/HD in the future."[10]

---

[10] Freeman, Roger D., M.D., "The Use of Stimulant Drugs in Attention Deficit/Hyperactivity Disorder Combined with Tics or Tourette Syndrome," 1994. Used with permission of the Tourette Syndrome Association, Inc.

Vacation from Medication?

At one time, "drug holidays" were recommended for youngsters on medication for TS and associated behavioral problems. The theory was that summertime was less structured and that there was less need to control tics or restrict inattention.

The majority of experts interviewed for this book, however, saw no reason to take a patient off medication providing (1) the patient was doing well with a minimum of side effects and (2) the patient was being properly monitored by a knowledgeable medical professional. A specific dosage can be reduced from time to time to determine if the minimal amount required to be effective has changed, but because of the waxing and waning pattern of TS, it's difficult to determine if less medication is needed or if a particular tic has just disappeared for a period.

If a medication is going to be discontinued, however, it should not be abruptly stopped, but rather slowly decreased, just as the new medication will be slowly increased.

How to Monitor Medications

As with any illness, a family quickly becomes fluent in the vocabulary of Tourette Syndrome. For those requiring medication to control tics and other problems, words like *Haldol, Orap,* and *Anafranil* come rolling off the tongue as easily as *aspirin* or *antibiotic* to the rest of the population.

But because no two people react to medication the same way, it's important to be knowledgeable about those prescription drugs. It's not enough to say, "It's the little white pill." Among the things you need to know about every pill you or your child takes are the following items:

1. The name of each particular medication
2. Its description
3. Why it is being prescribed
4. The exact dosage being prescribed
5. How it should be taken (e.g., at night, after meals)

6. Potential side effects
7. Any medicines or drugs (including alcohol) or foods that interact adversely with this particular medication
8. Length of time before the effectiveness of the medication is likely to be seen
9. Long-term effects of the medication

As all this is a great deal to remember, keep a notebook with this information. Note and date reactions or side effects as well as any positive effects. Record the date when dosage is altered and any resulting side effects.

Also list any events occurring on a particular date that might alter the medication's expected effect. For example, if your youngster is ill or anxious over a coming exam, the tics might increase in intensity or frequency. That information would assure you and the physician that the dosage was probably adequate, but that environmental influences were at work.

Never trust your memory. Write it down. Also include your questions concerning medications so you remember to ask at the next visit.

If you cannot find a physician in your community who is knowledgeable in dealing with these medications, contact the TSA for the names of experts nearest you. Often a family will go to a clinic specializing in the treatment of Tourette Syndrome for a consultation and prescription for medication, if needed, and then return home to work with their local professional. (Most physicians are willing to learn from their peers. It is difficult for them to be expert in all phases of all diseases and disorders. If your doctor is one of the minority who is not cooperative, find another who is.)

Alternative Therapies

Many of the symptoms of Tourette Syndrome—sniffing, throat clearing, nose twitching, and eye blinking—are also common to people suffering from allergies. In fact, some children displaying these symptoms often are first sent to an otolaryngologist or an allergist. Some of them actually may have allergies; others may have both allergies and TS; and still others may simply have TS with allergy-like symptoms.

Doris Rapp, M.D., pediatrician and children's allergist, and author of *Is This Your Child?* writes, "most physicians do not believe that allergy is in any way related to TS. It appears, however, that when some children's allergic symptoms respond favorably to allergy treatment, their manifestations of TS are also simultaneously relieved."

To the best of my knowledge, no replicated study of TS and allergy treatment has been conducted. Environmental medicine has identified some of the more obvious triggers for allergies— smoke, animal dander, molds, pollen, and certain chemicals. Continued investigation may lead to uncovering additional specific agents that may intensify symptoms of TS. If you think you or your child has a unique reaction to certain foods, seek out a professional nutritionist or allergist for treatment.

Hypnosis and biofeedback are two additional modalities of therapy for TS often mentioned when discussing alternative therapies. While there have been some documented cases of the severity and frequency of tics being lessened by these treatments, it is difficult to ascertain if the symptom reduction was, indeed, the effects of the biofeedback and/or hypnosis or the normal waxing and waning pattern of TS tics. It has been studied and proven, however, that both hypnosis and biofeedback are effective strategies for reducing stress and promoting relaxation, which in turn may prove beneficial in decreasing frequency and intensity of tics.

Although the TSA does not officially endorse any of the many alternative therapies tried for TS treatment, some professional and laypeople disagree. There is an Alternative Therapy Network where you can write to request their newsletter, "Latitudes," which offers information concerning ways claimed to reduce TS symptoms through nonpharmacological intervention. Enclose $2.00 for postage.

Alternative Therapy Network for Tourette Syndrome
P.O. Box 31256
Palm Beach Gardens, FL 33420-1256

At present, no magic elixir or miracle pill exists as a cure for Tourette Syndrome. While it's fine to learn about various treatments with proven success and duplicated in controlled studies, remember that desperate families and patients sometimes become unwitting targets for those who prey on such sorrow, promising a "quick fix." Be alert for such assurance and recognize that when a new proven treatment or cure is found, the TSA has the mechanism in place to inform us of it.

CHAPTER 6

Tracing the History

The history of Tourette Syndrome is an important and fascinating one. Understanding the history is vital because it demonstrates how easily false information can be transmitted and, in short order, become accepted as a universal truth.

The modern-day understanding of Tourette Syndrome had its beginning in the early 1800s, when the French neurologist Itard took as his patient a French noblewoman, the Marquise de Dampierre. She had become a recluse because of her bizarre symptoms that began when she was seven. In 1825, Itard wrote, "Thus in the middle of a conversation that interests her, suddenly without being able to avoid it, she interrupts that which she says or hears by bizarre cries and extraordinary words which make deplorable contrast to her distinguished manner." In addition, she displayed a variety of movements in her arms and hands, movements of her shoulder and neck, and the verbalizations—both obscene and nonsensical—of which he wrote.

Despite enjoying a brief eighteen- to twenty-month respite from her symptoms when she was seventeen, the Marquise de Dampierre continued to have coprolalia and other severe tics throughout her life until she died at age eighty-six.

Georges Albert Edouard Brutus Gilles de la Tourette (1857–1904), a protégé of the neurologist Charcot and a prolific writer, studied the case history of Itard's noblewoman along with two other cases involving similar bizarre symptoms. He considered the similarities in these and in six of his own patients, and in 1885, wrote a paper describing these findings. Gilles de la Tourette was the first to classify these people as suffering from a distinct disorder quite unique from other tic disorders. His mentor, Charcot, agreed and the new entity was named after Gilles de la Tourette.

Even in the mid-nineteenth century, Tourette believed the disorder now named for him to be hereditarily based. He also stressed that there was no intellectual or psychological deterioration. According to researchers Arthur Shapiro, M.D., and Elaine Shapiro, Ph.D., "Other factors identified by Tourette were its childhood onset, usually before puberty, the male predominance, and that the symptoms are progressive, with new ones added to or replacing old ones. He believed social class as well as geography to be of no importance because all social classes and people from many different areas were affected."

With the dawning of the twentieth century, however, came the age of psychoanalysis. New theories swirled like desert sand as psychiatrists and psychologists tried to find answers for the cause of Tourette Syndrome and its mystifying symptoms. Hysteria, schizophrenia, mental instability, sexual dysfunction, and narcissistic disorder were just a few of the explanations of that era. Poor family dynamics often were stressed, with the mother usually mentioned as the major villain.

It wasn't until the mid-1960s, with work done by researchers such as the Shapiros, Dr. F. S. Abuzzahab, and others that our present understanding of Tourette Syndrome came into being, one that finally acknowledged the disorder's biological basis, thus altering (hopefully forever) the belief that TS was a psychogenic disorder.

Educating others, however, is an ongoing process. Parents have described spending hours attempting to educate school personnel about their child's Tourette Syndrome, using the fine materials provided by the Tourette Syndrome Association, supportive articles from magazines, and even showing instructional films specifically created to help others understand Tourette Syndrome, only to have a principal or child's teacher nod, smile, and say, "Yes, but if Shelley would just try to keep from making those sounds in class she wouldn't be so disruptive."

I've experienced this resistance to understanding the truth about Tourette Syndrome firsthand as well. Those of us with a personal interest in TS need to know the facts in order to share them with others. There's still a great deal of educating to do.

CHAPTER 7

Making the Diagnosis

The techniques used to diagnose Tourette Syndrome—the taking of a careful and complete history and observation of symptoms—are, by their very nature, subject to error. Although medical students are usually taught in the second year of their studies how to take a patient's history, people, being human, are diverse and unique beings. Some physicians may be better listeners than others; some may instinctively know just how to phrase a question in order to elicit the best (i.e., most honest and complete) response. Others may be prejudiced and have their minds made up even before completing the history, or may be one of those (fortunately) rare breeds of physicians in a pediatric specialty or subspecialty who cannot deal with parents (especially mothers). It happened to me.

The year was 1972. My daughter, Leslie (not her real name), and I pressed against the back of an already cramped examination room at a major medical center to make way for the chief of pediatric neurology and a flock of male residents trailing behind him like baby ducks waddling after the mother duck.

He swooped in and turned to his followers with a flourish. "This woman," he said, with an intonation that made me cringe, "has brought this nine-year-old female to us with a complaint of nervous tics." He turned to me and added in a tone usually reserved for the infirm, the elderly, or the mentally incompetent, "Why don't you tell these gentlemen in your own words?"

I looked into their youthful faces, feeling I had already been judged and somehow found lacking. Nevertheless, I was Leslie's mother. I would present her case as carefully as I knew how.

"It began with a shrug . . . she'd shrug her shoulders. . . ."

"When?" the doctor interrupted.

"You mean in what situations would she do it?"

"No," he said, shaking his head in exasperation and raising his voice slightly. "When did she first begin the shrugging?"

I thought a minute. When? How do you know when a tic actually begins? You just notice that your child is doing it again.

"Well?" he demanded as though I was keeping them from an important appointment.

"Well," I said cautiously, fully aware that the residents had pens poised to record my answer. "I think the shrugging began about two years ago. . . ." They wrote that down. "But I can't be sure." They glared as a group.

"And then . . ." he prompted, looking at his watch.

"Then the shrugging went away . . . and she began blinking her eyes, then clearing her throat."

"Blinking? Clearing her throat?" he asked incredulously. Obviously he didn't consider these symptoms to be too serious.

I hurried on, despising the fact that I was so anxious to please that I searched to remember some symptom that they *would* find interesting.

"One thing led to another. She began sniffing, shaking her head, jerking her arm. . . ."

"All at once?"

"No, one tic would leave and another would replace it, although sometimes she'd have two or more."

"Anything else?" He picked up his clipboard and the residents capped their pens.

"Yes. She hooted. Barked really."

This well-known pediatric neurologist looked at me in disbelief. "Barked?"

"Barked." I dug in my handbag. "Here. I brought a tape recording of the sounds. So you could hear it. She doesn't seem to do any of these things when doctors are around."

For the first time, the physician looked at Leslie, as though she were some type of obscure specimen. "No," he said, smirking to the residents, "she looks perfectly fine to me. A normal little girl." My daughter sat silent, motionless, the antithesis of my description of her.

''Here's the tape,'' I said, thrusting it into his unwilling hands. ''Listen to it. You'll hear what I mean.''

Jamming the tape into the pocket of his white coat, he turned to the residents and smiled. ''Typical overwrought, overcontrolling, overeducated mother,'' he said. The physician patted me on the shoulder, turned, and led his solemn-looking troop out of the room.

It took us three additional years—years of heartaches, tears, and undescribable guilt—before my husband, daughter, and I found ourselves in the office of Arthur Shapiro, the New York City psychiatrist who diagnosed her as showing the classic symptoms of a neurological disorder known as Tourette Syndrome.

My story is not unique. Fortunately, today there are lightweight handheld video cameras so you can easily record your child's tics—both motor and verbal—without the youngster knowing your true purpose and thus becoming inhibited. Hopefully, *your* physician will be willing to watch the video. If not, find another who will.

Finding the Right Physician

It isn't realistic to assume, however, that every doctor in your medical insurance plan will necessarily know how to diagnose and treat TS. Even today there are physicians who are unaware of the disorder or who think there has to be coprolalia or echolalia present in order to make that diagnosis. If you can't locate a doctor who is knowledgeable about TS, call the TSA and ask for recommendations of physicians in your area as well as the names of those he or she has treated.

If the patient is your child, you'll need a pediatrician who can deal with your youngster's usual childhood ailments along with the TS and accompanying behavioral problems. In addition, the doctor needs a style of practicing that makes you feel comfortable. Doctors have different personalities just as patients do. It's in the best interest of your child that you and your child's doctor are a compatible match. Some people prefer doctors who are paternalistic and authoritarian, telling them what to do, while others want to be active participants, part of the team. Don't underestimate the importance of choosing the right physician for you and your child. You'll be working together for a long time.

It's just as important to make the right match when you're the patient. Don't create more stress in your life by "hiring" a doctor who makes you feel uncomfortable.

Gathering the Facts

At your first meeting with your pediatrician or neurologist, psychologist, or psychiatrist, remember that the value of the history you give depends on your giving honest and complete answers. This information may help to diagnose your child and, in many cases, you as well. Many parents first learn of their own Tourette Syndrome when their child is diagnosed.

Try to report your family history accurately. It helps if you've done some sleuthing beforehand and written down what you've learned. If everyone always said that Great Aunt Martha was a little eccentric, try to discover why. Did she say inappropriate things? Make unusual gestures? Did she have an obsessive routine of checking things, counting or lining items up just so? If you can't remember, ask a grandparent, older friend, or relative who may have known her. Often there is someone in the family who also had tics that may have been Tourette Syndrome.

You may have difficulty remembering when your own child began having tics too. It's human nature not to notice things until one day we think, "He's still doing that." Have a meeting with your spouse, friends, and other family members. Someone may point out that Junior's sniffling went on long after allergy season last year or that Katie continued to shake her head and make blowing sounds, even after you cut her bangs. The mind is selective. We don't always remember things just as they really were.

Use a video camera, tape recorder, or still camera to try to preserve the sight and/or sound of various tics. Don't assume that your child will "perform" in front of the doctor.

Try to stay focused on the subject. That's where making notes beforehand helps. Although the physician wants to help, time is always in short demand. Don't waste valuable minutes by saying, "I think it was Thanksgiving . . . no, it was Christmas because the dog had just died and we . . ." Be concise and organized, reporting factually what you have seen and heard. Encourage your youngster to express himself or herself as well. It's not your disorder. It's your child's. He or she will have to take charge of it.

Communicating with Health-Care Professionals

To be effective, communication requires more than talking. The person to whom you're talking must receive and understand the message—*your* message. Often we—doctors and other health-care professionals, educators, parents, and patients alike—think that we have gotten our message across, only to discover that the other person has either misconstrued what we have said or hasn't a clue.

It's everybody's fault. We nod our heads as the physician speaks. Our body language says, "Yes, I understand." But we don't. The professional's vocabulary may be unfamiliar; we may still be in shock after learning our child has something wrong, so our brain has shut down; or we may be embarrassed to admit that we don't understand, so we pretend we do because we don't want to appear stupid. The doctor thinks we all are on the same page so he or she continues talking, confusing us all the more.

The health-care professionals are just as much at fault. A recent study found that patients described their complaints for an average of only eighteen seconds before their physician interrupted. Doctors often have waiting rooms filled with people who must be seen, so they're under a time constraint and feel the pressure. We pick up on their nonverbal cues—facial expressions, eye contact (or lack thereof), body movements (such as checking their watch or door hugging as they seem ready to bolt the room). Soon our stress rate matches theirs.

In addition, often physicians, psychologists, social workers, and other health-care professionals feel most comfortable with their brand of medical dialect so they revert to those terms and acronyms in their explanations. We—the parents or patients—sit there silently nodding like those little wooden dolls with the bouncing heads, so the professionals assume, incorrectly, that we speak and understand their language.

Although they may ask, ''Do you have any questions?'' they seldom ask us to restate what we think we heard to determine whether or not we understood correctly. We seldom ask any questions because (1) we know they are rushed, (2) we don't know what to ask, and (3) we don't want to feel dumb, or worse, have them think that we are. So we shake hands and leave, unsure of exactly what we heard, with our version differing from that of our spouse or child. We're confused, frustrated, depressed, and lost.

These communication errors not only erect walls of misunderstandings between parent and physician, parent and child, spouses, and everyone else who is involved, but they also can create treatment delays, both of which can have significant repercussions, especially when dealing with a condition as varied and relatively unknown as Tourette Syndrome and the sometimes tagalong conditions of ADHD and OCD.

Improve Listening Skills

Miscommunication can be a major problem. Below are a few tips for *both* the health-care professional and the parent/patient in order to get the most out of a meeting with one another.

PARENT/PATIENT

1. Make an appointment rather than trying to catch the doctor or other health-care giver in the hallway. Hallways of hospitals, clinics, and offices are not conducive to the giving or receiving of information.
2. Give the health-care professional your *full attention*. That means leaving a baby or toddler with a sitter so you're not

distracted. If your child is with you and is hyperactive, or the tics interfere with your concentration, ask for some time alone with the professional. Perhaps the nurse or a member of the office staff can look after your youngster while you get information and ask questions. Then your child can be brought back into the room to receive the same material on his or her level of understanding.

3. If you don't understand, say so. No one will think you're stupid. Despite their years of training, few health-care professionals are skilled at mind reading. They have no way of knowing if you're lost if you don't speak up.

4. Take notes or use a tape recorder so you can recall later what you're hearing now. You're getting a great deal of new information. It's difficult to process it all at once.

5. Write down questions when you think of them so you don't forget. Most people develop ''white coat amnesia'' when they see the doctor. No question is stupid, but no question gets asked if you don't remember it.

6. Remember that the health-care professional has other patients just as anxious as you to get diagnoses and information. Be prepared and don't waste time.

7. Ask for the best time to call with problems or questions as well as when calls are returned. Some physicians schedule time midday while others wait until after office hours to return calls. Knowing this beforehand prevents miscommunication later.

8. Be honest in answering the health-care professional's questions. If asked whether anyone in the family suffers from hyperactivity or obsessive-compulsive disorder, for example, be truthful. This isn't curiosity or prying; it's the proper way to take a history and could be important in treating you or your youngster.

HEALTH-CARE PROFESSIONAL

1. Schedule adequate time so that you can give the parents/patient your undivided attention.

2. Communicate on the same level. Ask the parents/patient to sit down and then also sit down, preferably without a desk separating you. When you stand over people they feel intimidated and may not be as receptive or able to focus on what you are saying.

3. Look directly at the parents/patient as you speak. Don't fiddle with papers on your desk, your watch, etc.

4. Try to speak in lay language; if you use medical terminology, explain it.

5. Ask if there are questions, then pause. If there are none, you might answer an unspoken question by saying, "Many people don't fully understand . . ." or "Try telling me in your own words about Junior, so I'm sure I didn't leave something out" (not ". . . so I know you understood.")

6. When you need to end the interview, hand the parents and/or patient printed educational information (brochures, videotapes, and other materials are available from the TSA) to reinforce what you've already told them.

7. Include support system data—the names and phone numbers of educational specialists as well as parents and patients who have agreed to serve as lay advisors. I frequently receive calls from frantic parents whose children have just received the diagnosis of Tourette Syndrome and who seem to have forgotten everything they've just heard from the health-care professional. Once we begin talking—parent to parent—they relax and often interject with, "Oh, yes, now I remember the doctor saying that."

CHAPTER 8

Recognizing OCD, ADHD, and Other Related Problems

Although in the late 1800s the French neurologist, Charcot, was the first to classify impulsive thoughts as a part of TS, one hundred years later there still was little mention made of the related problems of Tourette Syndrome. Recognition of these emerged only in the mid-1980s, when researchers began to hear similar reports from parents: "He's always moving. A real wiggle worm. It wears me out. Yesterday we found him climbing on the roof." "She seems to be listening in class, but it's as though the information goes in one ear and out the other. Her grades are dropping. We're all frustrated." "He can't seem to control his temper. I don't know what sets him off, but he blows up at the slightest thing."

In the 1970s, when I first heard the words *Tourette Syndrome,* there were only a handful of men and women doing research on this disorder. Most of them were poorly funded and struggled to complete their studies so they could be published and of benefit to others. Those professionals who did see patients and who could accurately identify the disorder made the diagnosis of Tourette Syndrome. We—parents and children—learned about motor and vocal tics, but never dreamed that there might be more to it than that. How could there be? What we saw and heard was enough of a burden.

But at that time we, the parents, were basically isolated from one another. In major cities, such as New York, there were clusters of identified TS patients—so much so, in fact, that at one point the patient population was so skewed that it was thought that TS might possibly be a "Jewish disorder" (which it isn't). But in the rest of the United States, in small-town America, and in most of Canada, the majority of families struggled to cope with the effects of Tourette Syndrome in a relative medical vacuum. Not only did most of our local physicians have little or no knowledge of Tourette Syndrome, many of the ones who *had* heard of the disorder still labored under the erroneous conclusion that it was a psychological problem.

We felt abandoned. We knew of no kindred parents with whom to discuss and compare those "other problems," those additional difficulties that we never connected with TS. Our kid had tantrums? He must be frustrated because of the tics. Doing poorly in school? It obviously was due to a low self-image because of the tics. Compulsive about cleanliness? Must be a tic. Every question we asked of our spouse late at night in the dark, we also answered, but always in terms of the tics. Cause and effect. It seemed likely.

In January 1970, a father of a son who had just been diagnosed with TS wrote a letter to the *New York Post* asking for other families with children having the same disorder to contact him.

Five families responded to his letter. The father asked Dr. Arthur Shapiro, a psychiatrist, who then was one of the few physicians both diagnosing TS and using haloperidol as an investigatory drug in the northeastern United States, to contact his patients to see if any of them were interested in helping to form a Tourette organization.

Shapiro recalled, "Twenty-two of my thirty-four patients agreed to attend that meeting. There were twenty-seven of us in all who met June of 1971 at the Payne Whitney Clinic and Cornell Medical School to form the Tourette Syndrome Association (TSA)." Martin Levey, the father who had placed the ad, was elected as its first president. Today there are close to fifty chapters in the United States and Canada with more than 28,000 families as members. There are more than 40,000 on the mailing list. In addition, there are TS organizations in more than a dozen foreign countries.

As more cases of TS were diagnosed, many of the families clung together like survivors of an earthquake, comparing notes and finding some small measure of comfort when others reported comparable observations. Telephone friendships developed across the country, providing an emotional lifeline—offering hope and support; sharing hard data, such as the names of knowledgeable physicians and new therapies (some that were effective and others that were not); and serving as an information exchange for behavioral and learning problems that kept rearing their ugly heads.

This pattern of additional problems—obsessive behavior, attention deficits, learning difficulties, hyperactivity, sleep disturbances, self-injurious behavior, and uncontrollable tempers—began being reported among the informal TS telephone circles, then shared in a more formalized setting by the TS support groups being formed around the country and in Canada. At first, they were only whispered between concerned parents, but finding confirmation within the parent group, the information was shared with researchers who set to work. All but a few of the controlled studies agreed with what the parents already knew: There *are* additional related problems that *may* affect some of those with Tourette Syndrome, but that do *not* need to be present in order to make the diagnosis of TS.

The findings in numerous studies confirmed what the children's parents and teachers had observed in their homes and schools for years: that many individuals with Tourette Syndrome also have varying degrees of obsessive-compulsive traits. A genetic relationship was suggested. (These conclusions, however, are not universally accepted within the medical community.)

Researchers also learned that about 30–50 percent of those with Tourette Syndrome may have attention deficit disorder (ADD) either with or without hyperactivity. In some instances, people may have both OCD and ADHD in addition to their Tourette Syndrome.

Remember that an individual *can* have TS without any of these associated disorders, and that few people have all of them. They are listed only to make you aware of the possibility and to be alert for signs of these potential tagalong behaviors.

Obsessive-Compulsive Disorder

According to the OC Foundation, a nonprofit organization whose purpose is to educate, promote research, and offer service to those with OCD, obsessive-compulsive disorder "is characterized by recurrent, unwanted and unpleasant thoughts (obsessions), and/or repetitive, ritualistic behaviors, which the person feels driven to perform (compulsions). People with OCD know their obsessions and compulsions are irrational or excessive, yet find that they have little or no control over them."

Most of us have some type of compulsive behavior. When my children were babies, I checked them at night, which consisted of peering over the side of the crib to be sure they were breathing. If I didn't see their tiny chests moving, I'd poke at them until they moved in their sleep. Was that obsessive-compulsive behavior? No, because when my husband teased me about it, I was able to stop doing it without experiencing any anxiety.

Someone who truly had an obsessive-compulsive disorder would have felt an extreme need to keep checking and would have felt uncomfortable and extremely anxious if prevented from carrying out the compulsive activity even if he or she understood it was silly or unnecessary.

Compare this behavior to the more complicated anecdote shared by a woman I met at a recent national TSA conference. "I always fear that something's going to happen to my husband on his way to work," she said, "so I have to call him to be sure he's all right. As soon as we've hung up, I think, 'maybe a filing cabinet fell over on him and hit his head,' so I have to call him back, even if I know it's an unlikely occurrence. It makes him angry when I bother him like that, but I can't help it."

"Obsessive-compulsive disorder becomes a problem when it interferes in your life as mine does," a mailman said. "I have to leave for work early in order to be able to complete all my rituals. I'm obsessed with the number nine. I don't know why. I count the nines on every house I pass and have to walk in steps of three because they make nine. If I get somewhere and it doesn't add up to nine, I have to walk in a little circle to make it come out all right."

Other adults told of actually spending hours counting things. A housewife known as a compulsive cleaner by her friends admitted that they only knew a part of her secret. Like many with OCD, she hid the extent of her behaviors. "They'd think I was crazy if they knew," she said tearfully. According to Judith Rapoport, M.D., principal investigator of OCD at the U.S. National Institutes of Health, "People with OCD are the world's greatest actors and actresses because they hide their rituals so well."

This housewife was no exception as, according to her, neither her husband nor their three children had any idea that she had OCD. As soon as her family left home for work and school, she hurried to the bathroom where she compulsively scrubbed the tub with three different brushes and dried it with three separate rags. "I have to count the towels in the linen closet, the soap under the sink, even the extra rolls of toilet paper. If any of them end up as an even number, I have to go out and buy another so it's always an odd total. But when I get back, I have to start over with the tub and go through the entire ritual again. I know it's nutty but I can't help it." She also lines up shoes and hangers in the closet and dusts every bookshelf in the house, counting each book as she takes it off and lining each up exactly so when she puts them back. Each shelf also contains an odd number of books.

Does this exhausting ritual make her feel better? "Only for a short time," she admitted. "Then I have to do others. I have different rituals I do just before the kids come home. It's stressful knowing I have to complete everything before they walk in the door, but the timing's part of it. If they ever knew about my symptoms, I'd die of embarrassment."

Schoolchildren who have obsessive-compulsive disorder suffer more than humiliation. Their class work tends to deteriorate. These youngsters may rewrite a paper many times or make holes in it as they erase and erase, trying to make it flawless. Chances are they'll also miss a homework deadline because they can't force themselves to turn in a report that is less than perfect. They may have trouble taking notes in class because they count words over and over again, or miss out on entire lectures as obsessive thoughts fill their minds. They are late for school because they tie and retie their shoes until the bow is exactly right, insist on wearing the same shirt for days or changing clothes continually, wash their hands constantly or have to pack their gym bag in a precise manner. Their obsessive-compulsive behavior continually keeps them behind schedule, late for activities, and may make them the laughing stock of their peers.

The rituals that bring pleasure to others—celebrating holidays and birthdays, sitting in special seats around the family dinner table, even starting a new school year with brand new notebook, shoes, and first-day outfit—are potential avenues of torment for those with OCD because of the anxiety associated with any type of deviation. This often pits them against other family members and/or friends creating additional tension that intensifies the severity and frequency of their tics. But they stand firm. For them, the ritual is set in concrete and even the thought of change brings pain. The person with OCD knows that he or she is doing something inappropriate, but still cannot stop doing it.

This type of behavior can play havoc with social and family life, school and work relationships. Many families turn themselves upside down, trying to make allowances for the person with OCD and sometimes denying that the actions are in any way different. Usually, however, family and friends cannot understand why someone who compulsively counts to 7 seven times after hearing that number mentioned doesn't just stop doing it, or why the person who scrubs his hands until they bleed keeps engaging in such bizarre behavior. Usually, these individuals don't understand either. "I just have to do it," they explain helplessly, even though they know it seems strange. Studies reveal that often it is OCD and not the tics that make these individuals slow to mature socially and to often experience difficulty once they're adults, trying to create and maintain friendships and/or relationships.

There are a number of "typical" obsessions that seem to appear in people throughout the world. These include:

- Fear of dirt, germs, and contamination
- Fear of acting on violent or aggressive impulses
- Overconcern with order, arrangement, or symmetry
- Constant doubts

- Abhorrent thoughts that violate society's mores
- Feeling overly responsible for everything
- Saving and hoarding

As with TS, the symptoms of OCD tend to follow a waxing and waning course. This, along with the fact that those with OCD excel in masking their behavior, makes the diagnosis of OCD often somewhat more difficult to make.

Although OCD typically begins in adolescence or early adulthood, it also may emerge in childhood. According to the American Psychiatric Association, the diagnostic criteria used to determine OCD include:

A. Either obsessions or compulsions

Obsessions as defined by (1), (2), (3), and (4):

(1) recurrent and persistent thoughts, impulses, or images that are experienced, at some time during the disturbance, as intrusive and inappropriate and that cause marked anxiety or distress

(2) the thoughts, impulses, or images are not simply excessive worries about real-life problems

(3) the person attempts to ignore or suppress such thoughts, impulses, or images, or to neutralize them with some other thought or action

(4) the person recognizes that the obsessional thoughts, impulses, or images are a product of his or her own mind (not imposed from without as in thought insertion)

Compulsions as defined by (1) and (2):

(5) repetitive behaviors (e.g., hand washing, ordering, checking) or mental acts (e.g., praying, counting, repeating words silently) that the person feels driven to perform in response to an obsession, or according to rules that must be applied rigidly

(6) the behaviors or mental acts are aimed at preventing or reducing distress or preventing some dreaded event or situation; however, these behaviors or mental acts either are not connected in a realistic way with what they are designed to neutralize or prevent or are clearly excessive

B. At some point during the course of the disorder, the person has recognized that the obsessions or compulsions are excessive or unreasonable. NOTE: This does not apply to children.

C. The obsessions or compulsions cause marked distress, are time consuming (take more than 1 hour a day), or significantly interfere with the person's normal routine, occupational (or academic) functioning, or usual social activities or relationships.

D. If another Axis I disorder is present, the content of the obsessions or compulsions is not restricted to it (e.g., preoccupation with food in the presence of an Eating Disorder; hair pulling in the presence of Trichotillomania; concern with appearance in the presence of Body Dysmorphic Disorder; preoccupation with drugs in the presence of a Substance Use Disorder; preoccupation with having a serious illness in the presence of Hypochondriasis; preoccupation with sexual urges or fantasies in the presence of a Paraphilia; or guilty ruminations in the presence of Major Depressive Disorder).

E. The disturbance is not due to the direct physiological effects of a substance (e.g., a drug of abuse, a medication) or a general medical condition.

Specify if:

With Poor Insight: If, for most of the time during the current episode, the person does not recognize that the obsessions and compulsions are excessive or unreasonable.[1]

Another form of compulsion, *trichotillomania*, is difficult to keep successfully hidden from friends and family. It usually begins around puberty, at age twelve or thirteen. Those who have this condition feel that the only way they can relieve their anxiety is by pulling out their hair, either from their head or sometimes

---

[1] Reprinted with permission of American Psychiatric Association: *Diagnostic and Statistical Manual of Mental Disorders*, Fourth Edition. Washington, DC: American Psychiatric Association, 1994.

their eyebrows and eyelashes, pubic hair, or other body hair. Some actually pluck themselves bald and must resort to wearing a wig. Many individuals play with the hair once it is pulled out and some may even eat the entire strand of hair. According to the National Institute of Mental Health, it is estimated that there are 4–8 million people in the United States who suffer from this subtype of OCD, 90 percent of whom are female. Some researchers consider trichotillomania and other such symptoms of OCD to be a form of tics.

According to Dr. Judith Rapoport and others, psychoanalysis and traditional psychotherapy have not been particularly helpful forms of treatment for those with OCD. While talk therapy can help bolster self-image, along with other benefits, most studies suggest a possible genetic biochemical imbalance in the brain to be the cause of OCD. (As with TS, however, stress and other psychological factors may exacerbate the symptoms.)

Today, many people with OCD are being successfully treated with medications such as clomipramine (Anafranil), fluoxetine (Prozac), sertraline (Zoloft), paroxetine (Paxil), and fluvoxamine (Luvox), all drugs that act on the brain chemical or neurotransmitter known as *serotonin*. These medications are also used successfully in treating the depression that may sometimes accompany TS. As with the medications used in treating Tourette Syndrome, these prescription drugs need to be carefully balanced to achieve reduction of symptoms with a minimum of side effects.

All recent data indicate that the most effective intervention for OCD is medication plus behavior therapy. With this type of treatment, people are taught to first identify and then face their fears directly. Rather than performing the usual ritual to release the tension or anxiety that it creates, they are taught to use a new (and more acceptable) behavior or set of behaviors instead. Strong support by both the therapist and family is needed to help these individuals fight the urge to act on their compulsions in the previous manner. Unfortunately, behavior therapy appears to be successful with only about 25 percent of those suffering from OCD.

Taking part in a support group can often help someone with OCD by first underscoring that he or she is not the only one struggling with this condition, and by providing an additional community of caring and concerned friends to help strengthen the individual's resolve to succeed in the fight against his or her compulsions. A support group also acts as a social oasis for those whose OCD has kept them too busy ritualizing to learn basic socialization skills so that they can make (and keep) friends.

Some people with OCD have learned to make their disorder work for them, to some degree. Athletes, musicians, and dancers perfect their techniques through constant repetition of movement, while computer programmers, accountants, researchers, scientists, and artists utilize their intense concentration on details for greater success in their careers.

Learning how to deal with OCD is a book in itself and many outstanding ones have been written for families, friends, and coworkers dealing with this problem. A number of them are mentioned in the "Suggested Reading" section.

Attention Deficit Hyperactivity Disorder

This term is often used interchangeably with attention deficit disorder (ADD), hyperactivity, and minimal brain dysfunction (MBD). However, the two former disorders have different components and the latter, minimal brain dysfunction, is an older term from the 1960s and 1970s that is no longer used. It isn't that researchers couldn't decide what to call the disorder. Instead, it depends on what aspect of the disorder you are highlighting. For the purpose of this book, I prefer ADHD, as this is the disorder that is often found "traveling" alongside TS, although some individuals do not have a hyperactivity component.

Many people (percentages vary depending on which study is used) with TS also have attention deficit hyperactivity disorder, which causes them to be impulsive, restless, and inattentive. All these behaviors are destined to have negative effects on social interactions, learning abilities, and the psychological well-being for the child and adult alike.

As with much of medicine, there is not total agreement among researchers as to whether the gene responsible for TS also causes

ADHD, if having TS predisposes someone to ADHD, or if just having to cope with the severity of their tics makes people appear inattentive and impulsive.

According to Kenneth E. Towbin, M.D., and Mark A. Riddle, M.D., both of the Yale Child Study Center, "It is empirically evident that when children have more frequent and/or more forceful tics and other symptoms of TS it is more difficult for them to perform cognitively. Moreover, when the symptoms are more severe, it can be very difficult for children to contain many other impulses that arise in response to their involuntary loss of control. For some persons with TS, it may be that the capacities for attention, impulse control, and physical control are lower when compared to those of the general population, but not severe enough to warrant a clinical diagnosis of ADHD." They go on to say that "it is necessary to consider when symptoms of ADHD cause impairment in individuals with TS; whether the symptoms are 'comorbid,' 'secondary,' or a 'core feature' of TS, the patient is still suffering and in need of appropriate education, psychological, pharmacological, and family intervention."[2]

While environment and faulty parenting skills can make the symptoms worse, they do *not* cause ADHD. As with other neurological disorders, boys tend to show signs of ADHD in a 3:1 ratio with girls, although both sexes can inherit the tendency toward it. The telling symptoms of ADHD usually begin as early as four and almost always by age six, although many parents (mothers, usually) swear that they knew their child was hyperactive and had other problems from infancy.

One mother said, "They called from preschool and told me to come get him. He was two-and-a-half and was thrown out of play school, for God's sake. Not that I blamed them. He interrupted story hour, wiggled and hummed at rest time, and threw the blocks when the other kids wouldn't let him play with them. There were times I would have gladly given him away to the first

---

[2] Towbin, Kenneth E., and Mark A. Riddle, "Attention Deficit Hyperactivity Disorder," *Handbook of Tourette's Syndrome and Related Tic and Behavioral Disorders*, edited by Roger Kurlan (New York: Marcel Dekker, Inc., 1993).

person who asked.'' She paused, then added, ''This has *not* been a fun child.''

Unfortunately, these youngsters aren't fun for themselves either. They disrupt classrooms, frustrate and aggravate peers, pick fights, embarrass siblings, and often create tension between their parents. Experts in the field often are heard saying, ''With ADHD, it is 'Ready! Fire! Aim!' '' That speaks to the impulsivity or lack of impulse control that lands the person with ADHD into trouble at home, at school or work, and in social situations.

Attention deficit hyperactivity disorder is expressed by the person's inability to stay focused on a task, impulsivity, and/or excessive motor activity. But just as the symptoms of Tourette Syndrome may be vastly different from person to person, ranging anywhere from mild to severe, so are the expressions of attention deficit hyperactivity disorder.

As they did for both Tourette Syndrome and obsessive-compulsive disorder, the American Psychiatric Association has also listed symptoms, eight of which must be present for at least six months in order for the diagnosis of ADHD to be made.

A. Either (1) or (2)

(1) six (or more) of the following symptoms of **inattention** have persisted for at least 6 months to a degree that is maladaptive and inconsistent with developmental level:

Inattention

(a) often fails to give close attention to details or makes careless mistakes in schoolwork, work, or other activities

(b) often has difficulty sustaining attention in tasks or play activities

(c) often does not seem to listen when spoken to directly

(d) often does not follow through on instruction and fails to finish schoolwork, chores, or duties in the workplace (not due to oppositional behavior or failure to understand instructions)

(e) often has difficulty organizing tasks and activities

(f) often avoids, dislikes, or is reluctant to engage in tasks that require sustained mental effort (such as schoolwork or homework)

(g) often loses things necessary for tasks or activities (e.g., toys, school assignments, pencils, books, or tools)

(h) is often easily distracted by extraneous stimuli

(i) is often forgetful in daily activities

(2) six (or more) of the following symptoms of **hyperactivity-impulsivity** have persisted for at least 6 months to a degree that is maladaptive and inconsistent with developmental level:

Hyperactivity

(a) often fidgets with hands or feet or squirms in seat

(b) often leaves seat in classroom or in other situations in which remaining seated is expected

(c) often runs about or climbs excessively in situations in which it is inappropriate (in adolescents or adults, may be limited to subjective feelings of restlessness)

(d) often has difficulty playing or engaging in leisure activities quietly

(e) is often ''on the go'' or often acts as if ''driven by a motor''

(f) often talks excessively

Impulsivity

(g) often blurts out answers before questions have been completed

(h) often has difficulty awaiting turn

(i) often interrupts or intrudes on others (e.g., butts into conversations or games)

B. Some hyperactive-impulsive or inattentive symptoms that caused impairment were present before age 7 years.

C. Some impairment from the symptoms is present in two or more settings (e.g., at school [or work] and at home).

D. There must be clear evidence of clinically significant impairment in social, academic, or occupational functioning.

E. The symptoms do not occur exclusively during the course of a Pervasive Developmental Disorder, Schizophrenia, or other Psychotic Disorder and are not better accounted for by another mental disorder (e.g., Mood Disorder, Anxiety Disorder, Dissociative Disorder, or a Personality Disorder).[3]

There are other disorders with many similar symptoms of ADHD, so it is important for parents to seek help from a medical professional or health-care clinic with expertise in dealing with ADHD children.

As with Tourette Syndrome, there is, at present, no test—either physical or psychological—that can make a diagnosis of ADD or ADHD definite. It must be done by observation and the taking of a careful history. Again, similarly with TS, children often suppress symptoms of ADHD at the physician's office—sitting quietly with hands folded—much to the exhausted parents' amazement. It isn't that the youngster is necessarily being contrary. It is instead because these children *can* concentrate for short periods of time in certain situations. That's why parental and/or teacher diaries noting specific behaviors can be extremely helpful to the health-care professional.

Although there is medication that can help control ADHD in some individuals (see Chapter 5), there is, at present, no cure. The disorder can and usually does create numerous problems in school, personal, and business life.

Adults Have ADHD Too

Until recently, little was written about adults with ADHD because it was assumed, incorrectly, that someone with ADHD would eventually outgrow the condition. Unfortunately, studies now reveal that as many as 40–60 percent of children with ADHD will continue to have symptoms of it throughout adulthood, meaning that more than 10 million American adults today

---

[3] Reprinted by permission of the American Psychiatric Association: *Diagnostic and Statistical Manual of Mental Disorders*, Fourth Edition. Washington, DC: American Psychiatric Association, 1994.

may be struggling with the effects of ADHD. Even those whose TS tics have tapered off or become minimal as they approach their adult years may find their lives still complicated by the lack of self-confidence, diminished social skills, and difficulty in getting and holding a job because of their symptoms of ADD with or without hyperactivity.

"People understand my tics," a forty-year-old man told me, his fingers tapping out a frantic rhythm on the tabletop between us. "They knew I couldn't help yelping or banging my temples with my fists until I broke the nose piece on my glasses. What they couldn't accept—still can't—is that I'm impulsive, don't follow directions, and have this need to boss everyone. My frustration tolerance is nil and I know I overreact to things, but realize it only after I've already blown my top and it's too late to do anything about it. I don't mean to be the way I am. I can't help it. I know nobody likes me. I don't either." With that, he abruptly terminated the interview by jumping up and hurrying away.

In their book, *Driven to Distraction,* authors Edward M. Hallowell, M.D., and John J. Ratey, M.D., list what they consider to be "Suggested Diagnostic Criteria for Attention Deficit Disorder in Adults." It is as follows:

NOTE: Consider a criterion met only if the behavior is considerably more frequent than that of most people of the same mental age.

A. A chronic disturbance in which at least fifteen of the following are present:

   (1) A sense of underachievement, of not meeting one's goals (regardless of how much one has actually accomplished).
   (2) Difficulty in getting organized.
   (3) Chronic procrastination or trouble getting started.
   (4) Many projects going simultaneously; trouble with follow-through.
   (5) Tendency to say what comes to mind.
   (6) A frequent search for high stimulation.
   (7) An intolerance of boredom.

(8) Easy distractibility, trouble focusing attention, tendency to tune out or drift away in the middle of a page or a conversation, often coupled with an ability to hyperfocus at times.

(9) Trouble in going through established channels, following "proper" procedure.

(10) Impatient: low tolerance for frustration.

(11) Impulsive, either verbally or in action, as in impulsive spending of money, changing plans, enacting new schemes or career plans, and the like.

(12) Tendency to worry needlessly, endlessly; tendency to scan the horizon looking for something to worry about, alternating with inattention to or disregard for actual dangers.

(13) Sense of insecurity.

(14) Mood swings, mood lability especially when disengaged from a person or project.

(15) Restlessness.

(16) Tendency toward addictive behavior.

(17) Chronic problems with self-esteem.

(18) Inaccurate self-observation.

(19) Family history of ADD or manic-depressive illness or depression.

B. Childhood history of ADD

C. Situation not explained by other medical or psychiatric condition.[4]

Hallowell and Ratey stress in their book that people with ADD may nevertheless be creative, intuitive, and highly intelligent.

There's no doubt that many of us adults with TS also cope with varying degrees of ADHD and that there needs to be greater awareness among the public and medical communities that it does affect adults as well as children.

As with OCD, the problems relating to ADHD are numerous as are the solutions. I have listed a number of helpful books dealing with ADHD in the "Suggested Reading" section.

---

[4] Reprinted by permission. Hallowell, Edward M., M.D., and John J. Ratey, M.D., *Driven to Distraction* (New York: Pantheon Books, 1994).

Aggression and Tourette Syndrome

Some children and adults with TS also have difficulty in handling frustration and anger. They strike out at others and, in some instances, at themselves as well, hitting, kicking, biting, or throwing things. Whether this hostility and rage arises from the frustration and anger involved in dealing with Tourette Syndrome or has a biological cause is still unknown, although researchers are diligently tackling this issue.

Ways of handling these tantrums and often frightening expressions of anger are detailed in many of the books listed under "Suggested Reading." It's important to teach a youngster (or learn yourself, if you suffer from rages) that hurting others will not be tolerated. Relaxation techniques mentioned in Chapter 14 may be helpful along with "The ABC's Cooling-Off Tips," which include:

A = always keep your hands in your pockets
B = breathe in deeply and slowly let it out
C = count to 10
D = don't yell, tell (which is another way of saying "communicate your feelings")
E = edit your thoughts (like a movie editor focusing the camera on another, more peaceful picture)
F = find something else to do

You can continue on with the alphabet, although six points may be about all a person can handle at one time. Encourage exercise, as well, as it's difficult to be furious when you're race walking, swimming, or running.

Touching

Many people with TS admitted that they had a touching tic (compulsion?). For some, it was touching breakable objects in a shop, food at a grocery, or all the parking meters along the street.

The eighteenth-century writer Samuel Johnson was said to touch every post on the street as he walked. One man described touching paintings in various art galleries and setting off the alarm. Numerous individuals described having to even things up if they touched someone or something on one side by touching it on the opposite side. Others constantly touch and tug at their clothing and hair.

Some people with TS touch the ground with their hand as they walk, often masking it to look as though they were picking up a coin or a leaf. Others touch a book, coffee cup, silverware, or other objects with their nose or tongue.

More serious touching problems arise when the individual constantly touches his or her own breasts or genitals in public or grabs at a stranger's breast, buttocks, or genitals.

Another potentially dangerous touching behavior (also a type of self-injurious behavior) is touching hot stoves, electrical wires, or stray animals.

Smelling

Some people with TS have the need to smell things. They'll smell their shoes before putting them on or underwear after removing the items. They sniff at their fingers. At school or work they smell the paper, books, even their pencils. Out-of-doors, some individuals will bend down to smell the grass, pick leaves to smell, or even sniff at trees. Sometimes they'll go up to strangers and attempt to smell them or their clothing.

Self-Injurious Behavior

Self-injurious behavior goes by many names, including self-mutilation, self-injury, and self-destructive behavior. With medicine's propensity to acronymize, it is often referred to as SIB.

In 1885, Georges Gilles de la Tourette described self-injurious behavior in one of his patients with Tourette Syndrome, a young man with numerous head and neck tics. He said, "His mouth opens wide; when it closes again one can hear the teeth of both jaws gnashing violently. Quite often his tongue is caught between them and abruptly seized and lacerated.'' According to several biographies on Dr. Samuel Johnson, he cut and picked at his fingernails until they bled.

Other self-injurious tics found in a minority of those with Tourette Syndrome include biting the lips or insides of the cheeks until sores form, licking the lips until they are chapped and crack, banging the head, hitting various parts of the body (on oneself or others), jabbing a finger against a hard object, placing fingers or the entire hand against the hot burner on a stove, poking at oneself with a pencil or other sharp instrument, sticking straight pins or needles into the skin, and injuring the eyes.

Dr. Roger Freeman admitted that self-injurious behavior (SIB) can be difficult to treat. ''We see more of it in a clinical sample than you might in the TS community at large,'' he said. ''But it is a significant problem when it occurs. Some people will pound on an existing bruise. Others will 'even it up' on the other side. We see patients who push and poke on their eyeballs, saying there is a 'feeling' behind it. They claim the pressing helps to create a sensation that relieves the pressure. In a few cases, they've seriously injured their eyes.''

One study based on questionnaires sent to members of the Tourette Syndrome Association in the United States resulted in 111 responses. Of that number, 43 percent reported having ''SIB, of which the most common were head-banging, biting of the tongue, cheeks, lips, and extremities, and self-hitting.''[5]

To informally test those results, I made some inquiries myself. Ten of fifteen individuals with TS admitted that they had, at some time, injured themselves on purpose. They described it as a loss of impulse control.

''I cut myself on my face with a razor,'' a young woman said. ''I didn't cut deeply, just enough to break the skin and make it

---

[5] Robertson, Mary May, and Jessica W. Yakeley, ''Obsessive-Compulsive Disorder and Self-Injurious Behavior,'' *Handbook of Tourette's Syndrome and Related Tic and Behavioral Disorders* (New York: Marcel Dekker, Inc., 1993).

bleed. I can't tell you why I did it. I just . . . had to." When asked how her parents had responded, she laughed. "I just told them a neighbor cat had scratched me. They never asked what neighbor or what cat."

A young man said that during his high school years he repeatedly hit himself on the upper cheekbone hard enough to blacken his eye. "My excuse was that I had run into a door. No one ever wondered why I was so awkward that I kept running into doors. It wasn't that I liked the pain; I just felt compelled to hit myself there. After a few smacks, the urge dissipated. After a year or so, that tic went away and has never come back. I didn't know anyone else did that sort of thing until now, when you told me. I wish I had known then. I thought I was crazy."

Those with SIB often will pick at a scab until it bleeds or becomes infected. It is so prevalent that Dr. David E. Comings, director of the Tourette Syndrome Clinic and Department of Medical Genetics at the City of Hope National Medical Center, said, "I have a rule that any skin lesion in a TS patient is self-induced until proven otherwise."

Fortunately, Haldol seems to be effective for many with SIB, but the doctor has to know about the behavior before he or she can medicate for it.

Sleep Disorders

In the 1970s and early 1980s it was stated that those with TS did not tic in their sleep and some physicians still incorrectly assume that to be true. However, more recent findings have altered the thinking. Although there have been few controlled studies concerning sleep and TS, a 1983 monitored sleep study conducted by Drs. Daniel G. Glaze, James D. Frost Jr., and Joseph Jankovic of Baylor College of Medicine in Houston demonstrated that their subjects did have motor tics during sleep, along with disturbed sleep patterns.

David E. Comings, M.D., also found that various sleep disturbances were prevalent among his TS patients, including difficulty in falling asleep; early waking; sleep walking; night terrors (where a child wakes up screaming, is difficult to arouse, and has no memory of the event in the morning); bed wetting (medically called "enuresis"); and sleep apnea, where a person briefly stops breathing during sleep.

Fortunately, it is highly unlikely that any one person will have all of the above problems that seem to be related in some way to Tourette Syndrome. They are mentioned only to bring the possibility to your attention, so that if you, your spouse, friend, or child demonstrates any of the above behaviors, you will know that others with TS have experienced them as well. Always discuss any behavioral change with your physician. There are medications that can help a number of these associated difficulties.

Part III

HOW TOURETTE SYNDROME AFFECTS A FAMILY

CHAPTER 9

Reacting to the Diagnosis

It's unlikely that you and your family will remain unchanged after learning that one of your family members has Tourette Syndrome. In fact, it's probable that you all were affected long before the diagnosis, both because of the waxing and waning nature of the TS symptoms, as well as because of the way in which the symptoms are expressed. Any chronic illness, because of the fact that it is chronic, changes family dynamics. Needs, expectations, and responsibilities are all altered with chronic illness, sometimes subtly, occasionally rather dramatically.

The true test of any family's functioning, however, develops when a family struggles to overcome adversity, conflicting diagnoses, and bewildering illness. In the process of learning to cope, the members frequently forge a unique strength and sense of closeness. Family members, challenged to find peace and purpose among chaos, often are amazed to find undiscovered resourcefulness and caring. Even the younger members usually prove themselves to be quite able to handle greater responsibility and are even pleased to be needed.

Too often, when there is illness in the family—a grandparent suffering a stroke, a loved one with cancer or AIDS (acquired immune deficiency syndrome) or even a sibling with emotional problems—most parents opt to protect their youngsters with a code of silence and shoo them away so they won't be frightened (or in the way). This is unfortunate because children, even those who are under five years of age, can learn to help care for those who are sick, and by doing so they get the message that they are important to the family and needed by the other members. This provides them with a vital sense of confidence and bolsters self-image, something every kid needs.

Handling the Diagnosis

There was so little known about TS when our first child was diagnosed that I think both my husband and I felt a great sense of relief that (1) she wasn't crazy; (2) we weren't lousy parents; (3) what she had actually had a name; and (4) there was something that could be done about it (i.e., medication to control some of the tics). We, of course, were not aware at that time that TS was a genetic disorder and that eventually two more of our children would be diagnosed with TS as well. We also didn't know how bad some of her tics would become before they finally tapered off and virtually disappeared, hopefully forever.

Some parents, however, feel no relief at all. I am on call to neurologists, psychiatrists, and pediatricians in my area to offer lay advice and support to families and children who have been newly diagnosed with Tourette Syndrome. Often a parent expresses bitterness and anger. "Why *my* child?" the mother or father will cry over the phone. "Why are we being punished?" I usually respond with what I learned from Rabbi Harold Kushner's book *When Bad Things Happen to Good People* and say that there's no answer; it's just bad luck.

In addition, these parents are mourning a type of loss of their child. The "perfect" child we all dream about is lost to them. They need time to grieve for that child, for others they hoped to have or do have (who may be similarly affected), and for themselves. Grandparents will often admit to feeling a sense of sadness for their child, their grandchild, and for themselves as well.

Also, there are additional reactions. Some parents deny that their "perfect" child could have a neurological problem and insist that they just need to become stricter (or less strict) in order to stop the tics. When the normal waxing and waning pattern makes the symptoms disappear for a while, it seems to support their viewpoint. Thus, valuable weeks, months, and even years may be wasted while parents continue to deny the diagnosis, and thus deny their child the very medication and emotional support that could help.

There are parents who keep the diagnosis a secret, even from the child. They continue to refer to the tics as "your habits" and excuse vocalizations as a "cough" and the head jerking as a "stiff neck." Their refusal to share the information with teachers, grandparents, and siblings makes it harder for the parents to cope and more difficult for the child to learn to live with a chronic condition, and hampers the efforts of teachers who might otherwise work with the youngster's problems if only they knew what was wrong.

Some parents feel resentment and envy that their relatives and friends have "normal" children. You may find yourself withdrawing or losing interest in others who don't seem to have problems with their youngsters. This is a normal reaction, one that you will probably overcome. If not, however, share your feelings with a qualified therapist or mental health counselor. Continued unresolved anger can hurt you, your marriage, and your child. Often, in this type of situation, the child with TS becomes the family's scapegoat, blamed for whatever misfortune visits the home.

Sometimes, one parent has a harder time adjusting than the other parent. This can create misunderstandings and tension between the couple just at the time when they need to comfort one another and work as a team. Open communication, which means talking freely and honestly about your feelings, fears, and frustrations, is vital. So is listening to your partner.

When the parents are divorced, the diagnosis of TS may become a battering ram to punish the former spouse. "He wouldn't have gotten this if you had been a better parent" is the refrain often used and equally painful to either the custodial parent or the noncustodial one. Each hurls accusations at the other, forgetting the frightened and ever-so-vulnerable child cowering between them.

A mother of a ten-year-old told me she felt no relief from her son's diagnosis. "It was better when we didn't know what it was," she insisted bitterly. As we talked, I learned that she still felt that TS must really be a mental disorder, and she was embarrassed to tell her parents and the other relatives that her child was mentally ill. When I explained that TS was caused by a chemical imbalance in the brain—that it was a neurobiological problem, not an emotional one—she finally seemed convinced. It wasn't that her child's physician hadn't told her exactly the same thing, but she had still been in shock then and probably hadn't heard much of what the doctor had said. That's why it's so important to take notes, ask questions, and read the materials made available through the Tourette Syndrome Association.

It's also a good idea to include the entire family—mother and father as well as the siblings—at that first meeting with the doctor after it is determined that the child does have TS. Often the mother and the affected child are the initial ones to hear the diagnosis. By the time they relay the information to the father, siblings, and extended family, some of the facts may be altered, much like what happens during the children's game of telephone.

There are numerous advantages to having a family conference with the physician.

1. Everyone hears the identical information at the same time (even though each individual may still interpret what he or she hears differently).
2. Each family member has the opportunity to ask questions that illustrate personal concerns or bias. For example, a sibling may ask if Tourette Syndrome is "catching" or if he or she could have "caused" the sibling to get TS, while a parent may wonder how a layperson keeps track of medication needs or how the disorder will affect future educational plans for the child.
3. Mother has visible support from the family and isn't thrust into the position of sole or main caregiver, a situation that often creates tension between spouses as well as adversely affects family dynamics.
4. Siblings feel that they are an important part of the support group, which helps them to cope with normal feelings of guilt (that they don't have TS) or jealousy (that the sibling with TS gets the majority of the parental attention).

5. The physician has the opportunity to see family dynamics at work, which is important because the family usually is the most vital support system for a child with Tourette Syndrome.

While some physicians may not feel comfortable in counseling families when they detect problem areas in family communication skills (sadly, it is an expertise not taught in most medical schools), hopefully they will refer family members to those social services or support groups in their community that have such expertise. In many cases, the local TS support group successfully serves this function.

It is essential that these families have the opportunity to learn "safe" methods of sharing their feelings and concerns so that they can be dealt with before additional stresses are created.

Stress and tension often make us speak without thinking. This is especially so when a new and seemingly more devastating tic appears. Become aware of emotional buildups and during those times think about what you're saying to those you love.

Avoid blaming one another for new tics. Shouting "I told you to get his hair cut" may make you feel better, but the truth is, your child will probably continue to shake his head and blow the nonexistent hair out of his eyes even after a haircut.

If you and your spouse disagree with house rules or other child management techniques, discuss it privately, not in front of the children. Avoid name calling, becoming defensive, or walking away. Turn off the television, turn on the telephone answering machine, and really listen to each other. Listen without thinking about what you're going to say next. Express what you're feeling. Strong communication skills can be developed with practice and are the cement holding a good marriage together.

If you haven't learned "fair fighting" rules, check your library or bookstore for self-help books or ask a mental health counselor for instruction. Take a course in assertiveness training at your local "Y," church or synagogue, or community college. These skills will permit you to express yourself without becoming aggressive.

A family quickly learns that a chronic illness such as Tourette

Syndrome has a rippling effect on many facets of family life. Parents considering a job change must now weigh the opportunities and possible raise in income against the difficulty of dealing with a probable change of insurance company and physicians. A move to a new community brings with it the additional need to reeducate the school personnel as well.

Some parents—particularly those in the public eye—may try to shield their youngster with TS from social or business situations that may be potentially embarrassing to the child (or to the parents). This can create resentments from siblings who are also banned, or guilt if they are included. For the child with TS, being left out becomes a reaffirmation that he or she is not okay.

Still others may react to the diagnosis by avoiding social and church or synagogue activities, in an effort to be there for their child. This type of smothering reinforces the youngster's lack of self-confidence and communicates the message that he or she must really be sick.

Don't expect everyone in the family to react the same to the diagnosis of Tourette Syndrome. In addition to having concern for the person with TS, it is normal to also have some apprehension about what this means on a personal level.

A sibling may react lovingly and be supportive, but at a deeper level may feel abandoned by the parents' total focus on the child with Tourette Syndrome, concern for what his or her peers may think, and fear that he or she in some way may have caused these tics. If the child with TS has behavioral problems as well, the sibling may feel real anger or resentment for all the tension and turmoil they create. There also may be a very real and underlying fear of "Will I get TS too?"

A father may feel shut out by his spouse's overprotectiveness toward the child with TS and worry about the future of his marital relationship as well as mourn his former warm father-child relationship. There may be concerns about the extra financial burden imposed by medications and additional doctor visits. He may fear that he appears less manly in the eyes of his peers because of his child's most visible disorder.

A mother may feel guilty for giving birth to a "defective" child, resentful that the burden of care has been dumped on her, and overwhelmed by the information concerning medications and their potential side effects. Additional demands by her other children, responsibilities for elderly parents, job, and housework, and lack of personal time may become physically exhausting, leaving her vulnerable to illness. She may tire of having to run interference for her child at school and of the need to become, as one mother called it, "educator to the world."

Adjustment to the diagnosis of TS does not magically appear overnight. Learning and then accepting that your child has a chronic condition is tough. It takes some people longer than others, but this acceptance is vital for everyone's well-being. You will have many questions. We did and still do. We also still look around at other children and young people at times and silently wonder, "Why *my* kid?"

Your reaction to the diagnosis of Tourette Syndrome, whatever it may be, is uniquely yours. There is no right or wrong way to react. You also may react differently at varying times, feeling bitter and resentful when your best friend complains about her kid's mild allergy problem, depressed when you think what lies ahead, hopeless and helpless as you see all the demands on your time and energy. Acknowledge and accept your feelings and move on. There's a great deal you need to know in order to help yourself and your child. It's nobody's fault; there's no guilt to assign.

Fortunately, others have marched before you. There are established information and support groups for you to access. Don't be afraid to ask for help. We've all been adrift and needed a life preserver to hug. Please contact:

The Tourette Syndrome Association
42–40 Bell Boulevard
Bayside, NY 11361-2820
(718) 224-2999
<tourette@ix.netcom.com>

This national organization has led the way in lay and professional education. In addition to working with local TS groups, they provide resource material for families, physicians, educators, etc. They can give you the number of your local TS chapter.

YOUR STATE OR LOCAL TS CHAPTER

Composed of families of those with TS as well as children and adults with Tourette Syndrome, this group can answer your questions concerning local services and organizations that can be helpful. Support groups meet on a regular basis, offering a chance to share information and feelings with other parents, siblings, and those with Tourette Syndrome. You are not alone.

NATIONAL AND REGIONAL CONFERENCES

The TSA sponsors both national and regional conferences. The 1993 National Conference in Houston was attended by 54 percent newcomers who not only heard international researchers discuss what was happening in the field of TS in terms of treatment, genetic studies, etc., but also had the opportunity to meet in workshops with others who live with Tourette Syndrome. While some parents with children having mild cases admitted to being overwhelmed by the severity of some of the attendees, most of those I interviewed expressed relief in meeting so many people who were coping well with the disorder.

COMPUTER NETWORKING

Those with computers and modems can communicate with others interested in TS through CompuServe's Health Forum and Prodigy. At this writing, CompuServe's TS group is found by first accessing the ADD forum. For Prodigy's TS forum, jump "medical" and then select "neurological." There are a number of subjects including "TS and drugs," and "TS and schooling." America Online and Delphi also have bulletin boards; they can be accessed at Usenet: <alt.support.tourette>

CHAPTER 10

Dealing with the Guilt

Although no one should feel guilty upon learning that his or her child has TS, many people do. After all, it's usually genetic. That means we must have "given it" to our child. How could we have done such a thing? The shock of knowing that we may have unknowingly hurt our child is unbearable. It's similar to the pain mothers of boys with hemophilia feel, needing to deal with the fact that they were the unwilling and unknowing carrier of their son's disease.

But many of us had kids never knowing that we might be carrying a gene that could cause TS in our children. We may or may not have had tics ourselves. Some may have full-blown Tourette Syndrome, but scientists weren't certain of the genetic link until recently, in about the last decade.

Now that we know about the genetic link, couples with a family history of TS must decide whether or not to have children or additional children. Most people I interviewed felt the risk was worth it. An advertising executive in the Midwest put it this way:

"I have a mild case of Tourette Syndrome. I knew that my children had a chance of inheriting the gene, and possibly might have TS as well. My wife and I discussed things before she got pregnant. One, our kids might not receive the gene; two, even if they did and actually had TS, it might be mild as mine is; three, even if it weren't as mild as mine, we felt we could handle whatever we were given. We knew we had a lot to offer children and we wanted them."

This couple eventually had two children. One has a mild case of TS and the other is free of any signs of TS or the accompanying disorders.

Two couples I interviewed had decided against having children since each couple had a parent with TS. Later, they changed their minds and decided to take their chances. "We have many talents and other 'good' genes for the kids to inherit too. If TS comes along in the package, we'll work with it. After all, we're experts by now."

A young woman in her early thirties thought differently, however. "My TS is most severe. I knew I didn't want to risk having a child with TS. When I was thirty, I had a tubal ligation. I've never regretted my decision."

The point to remember is that through your genetic pool you offer your children many things that are good and positive. If TS comes along with artistic skill or a wonderful personality, don't waste energy feeling guilty. It was not within your power to prevent it.

As the genetic component of Tourette Syndrome wasn't known when I had my children, my strongest feelings of guilt and regret for my actions stemmed from how we handled things during the prediagnosis years. Along with dragging our child to practically every type of medical specialist (doing the "doctor drag," we called it), trying to learn why she was doing these strange movements and sounds, we also resorted to bribery and frequent pleadings for her to stop. Sometimes I wondered if I was being punished for some misdeed in my life.

As we fortunately had a good relationship with our daughter, we never considered that she was acting out hostilities, although a psychologist once suggested that perhaps I was a "hovering mother" and she was reacting to my parenting skills (or lack thereof) by ticcing. I was particularly sensitive to that accusation, because as a parent, you want so much to make your child happy. It's tempting to try to intercede—to invite other children over to play, to call the ones who tease "dumb," and to want to make things better. Then you realize that you can't. You won't always be there to buffer your child against the world. That makes you feel guilty too.

Other parents have confessed to spanking or hitting their children to get them to stop ticcing, threatening to take away privileges, or sending them to their room until they can "get control of themselves." Some parents become so frustrated that they resort to verbal, emotional, and/or actual physical abuse.

Once parents understand that the child wants desperately to stop the tics but cannot, a wave of guilt may descend and continues each day as the tics remind you that you can't kiss it and make it go away, that you are powerless to help your child.

"I feel so guilty," a father admitted. "When I take my boy to movies or sporting events, people turn around to stare at his tics. I get angry at them, feel helpless that I can't do anything, and end up yelling at him. I must be an unfit father."

He isn't, of course.

Ask yourself, "What does my feeling guilty achieve? Does it make my child tic less? Does it make any of the accompanying behaviors less prominent? Does feeling guilty make *me* feel any better?" No? Then actively ban it from your emotional repertoire. Guilt leads to anger and depression, two additional burdensome emotions.

Practice using "Thought Stopping" techniques when you find yourself feeling angry when people stare at your youngster at the grocery or you see him or her ticcing in your home videos. Tell yourself, "Stop." Force yourself to refocus your mind on a pleasurable scene—your youngster laughing as he or she plays in the surf or sitting with you watching a beautiful sunset. You can't think of two things at once, so change your thoughts to those that make you feel good, not guilty. Don't suffer pain needlessly. It is within your power to change your thinking.

Remind yourself that many child experts, medical professionals, and others also were mistaken and/or ignorant about the nature of TS despite all their years of education and training. Your job is now, today, to love, support, and encourage your child with Tourette Syndrome. Remember too that the majority of children with TS lead normal and happy lives. They need supportive parents, not guilty ones.

CHAPTER 11

Coping with the Tics

One article I read on Tourette Syndrome advised parents to "just forget about the tics." It made me laugh. Obviously that writer had never listened to a child yelping, sniffing, grunting, or shouting obscenities during most of his waking hours. It's impossible to shut out the sounds regardless of how used to them you may be.

It is important, however, to avoid focusing on the tics. The more you frown at your child or put your finger to your lips to hush the sounds, the more stress you're adding, which makes it more likely the tics will become worse.

At Home

Home is supposed to be your child's safety zone, the one place where he or she doesn't have to suppress the tics, where the sounds and movements can freely be released in an atmosphere filled with love, understanding, and security. While it's impossible to forget about the tics, you and the rest of the family can learn to accept them as part of your child's unique extra baggage, just as you accept another child's wheezing from asthma, your spouse's limping from arthritis, or your parent's hearing aid.

There's no doubt that vocal tics are harder to ignore than the motor tics. They may, for example, make it difficult for the rest of the family to enjoy watching television. The youngster with TS may repeat what's being said or make noises that interfere with everyone else's concentration. Some families use individual headsets so they can watch programs with everyone present while others invest in a second television set, giving family members the option to watch their show in another room. You also might look into the wireless system used by many theaters for the hearing impaired.

As each tic is different, each brings with it different problems for the person with TS as well as for the family. Tics that may hurt or injure obviously must be dealt with at once. A tic that causes an arm to swing out, for example, may result in someone being hit or, as one mother reported, her child's fist hitting a mirror and shattering it, cutting her son's hand in the process.

"We learned the hard way to put away vases, picture frames, and other breakable objects that he may knock over," she said. "I can't take him shopping for fear he'll break a display case or knock over a mannequin. When he's around the baby, he tries—and usually succeeds—in substituting a different tic like waving his hand or holding his hands together."

Some individuals have self-injurious behavior (see Chapter 8), which is a difficult symptom to handle. Often it's hard to discern if an injury was accidental or SIB.

Many with coprolalia have learned to mask or substitute their vocal tics by saying "Fine" or "Full" or "Sure" and "She" rather than the obscenity. Substituting a different tic also may work with spitting or biting tics, although people vary in their ability to consciously change a tic even though they understand that their particular tic is potentially dangerous or offensive to others. Ask your child if the tic can be altered to a safer or more socially acceptable form. If not, and it does pose potential danger to the person with TS or others, seek help from a professional knowledgeable in treating TS. There are medications that often can minimize this type of tic.

Dealing with Strangers

Coping with the tics outside the home is far more difficult because it involves people who don't know anything about Tourette Syndrome and many who don't really want to know.

Some may feel threatened by the symptoms. "What would *you* think if you were shopping and saw a man rolling his eyes, showing his teeth in a weird grin, and grunting?" asked a middle-age man who displayed those very tics. "You'd probably grab onto your purse, avert your eyes, and cross the street."

It's difficult to anticipate the reactions of others. One young man reported working out in a gym. One of the forms his coprolalia took was muttering racial slurs, in this case, "nigger."

"I was so focused on exercising," he recalled, "that I didn't notice a big black man walking over to me. Everyone in the gym froze. I looked up, and there he was. 'Hey man,' this fellow said. 'Do you have that Tourette thing?' I told him I did. He asked me a few questions about it, then returned to what he was doing. Now, every time I go to the gym, he says 'Hi.'"

Everyone must determine how to handle this type of predicament. Each situation is so different, there's really no all-purpose way to handle things. If people stare at your child while you're standing in line at the grocery, you can (providing you and your youngster are both comfortable in doing so) say quietly, "He can't help making those noises. He has a disorder called Tourette Syndrome." Typically, some people will nod and say, "Oh, that's too bad." Others will just keep on staring. And, yes, there probably will be some who will sniff and respond with, "I think he just needs a good whack on the behind." An alternative to trying to explain (and to help educate) is to do nothing, to just act as though there is nothing out of the ordinary going on—which for you and your family is true.

If you're an adult with Tourette Syndrome, you may sense that strangers act as though they're a little afraid of you when they see and hear you doing your tics. Some people with TS (I've never been comfortable with the term "Touretter" as it sounds as though Tourette Syndrome is the individual's main identity) avoid eye contact, while others look directly at people and smile (as if to underscore that they are not dangerous or crazy). Some briefly apologize for their tics.

Still others purchase Medic Alert bracelets or necklaces that describe their symptoms, which may be important if the police or other law enforcement officers become involved for any reason.

For information about these identification bracelets and neck-laces, which come in stainless, sterling silver, or gold, contact Medic Alert, 1-800-344-3226, or write to them at P.O. Box 1009, Turlock, CA 95381-1009.

Unless you feel uncomfortable doing so. I think it is beneficial (to both strangers and yourself) to say to those standing closest to you, "I'm sorry if this bothers you. I have Tourette Syndrome." One young woman told me she had a printed card that she handed to strangers who stared. Many of them responded with, "Oh, yeah, I saw something about that on television."

Your response, of course, must be a little different when you attend a public performance. While vocal and motor tics blend right in with the way almost everyone else behaves at most sporting events (other than golf and tennis tournaments) or rock concerts, they could be very disruptive at ballets, symphonic concerts, plays, or movies. Most families plan "escape routes" so the person with TS can slip out and go to the restroom or lobby to release the symptoms.

While some families rely solely on videotapes for viewing movies and concerts at home, I personally believe hiding out serves only to accent an individual's sense of isolation. There are weeknights, afternoon, and other off-time showings of most movies that draw smaller audiences, which may be less stressful for the person with TS and therefore less likely to trigger additional tics. Try this approach from time to time before giving up entirely on going out to the movies.

Going out to restaurants presents another difficult situation for families with Tourette Syndrome, especially if there's a hyper-active component as well. In addition to the phonic tics, the person with TS may inadvertently fling dishes off the table, knock over water goblets, and spit out food. Hyperactivity may make it difficult for the person to stay seated and wait for the food to be served. In addition to making dining stressful for the person with TS and the rest of the family, these symptoms create an unpleasant atmosphere for the other restaurant guests.

Does this mean that a family with a member having Tourette Syndrome is forever doomed to ordering in or using the drive-through line? Not at all. It does, however, encourage careful selection of restaurants and the time of the reservation. Many restaurants have private rooms that you can request for no additional charge. You also can order ahead so there is less of a wait for the food to be served. And by going earlier than most diners, you'll find the restaurant less crowded (and the food often less expensive), which again means a less stressful situation for someone with TS.

Never tell a child with Tourette Syndrome that he or she can go out for dinner (or to the movies, ballet, etc.) with a promise to try to keep from making noises or wiggling. It puts an impossible burden on someone with TS. The stress it inflicts is both overwhelming and unfair.

Remember that fatigue tends to intensify tics, so if your plans include dinner and/or an outing, be sure the person with TS feels adequately rested. The day of exams or after coming home from a long trip may not be the time to plan such activities. Listen to your youngster. If he or she doesn't feel up to being in a public place, don't force it. People with Tourette Syndrome usually know what they feel capable of at a given time. You wouldn't force those with diabetes or asthma to do more than they felt up to, would you?

Dental and Medical Procedures

People with TS have to cope with the same dental and medical issues as those without the disorder. It just presents more of a challenge and an opportunity for creative solutions for those with TS.

A person with a head jerk, shoulder shrug, or teeth biting or grinding tic or who has hyperactivity may find it difficult to sit still long enough for routine teeth cleaning, application and adjustment of braces, cavity and root canal work, or periodontal surgery. Always discuss the problem with the dentist *before* he or she begins to work. Some individuals described being able to suppress the tic while the dentist worked, while others preferred the use of a mild sedative. The TSA has names of a few dentists who have treated individuals with TS. Also check your nearest major medical center or medical school.

Individuals requiring injections, blood tests, endoscopy or other invasive exams, glaucoma testing, or contact lens fitting—any medical treatment requiring one to remain motionless for a period of time—also should discuss their tics with the health-care professional in advance so that extra time can be allotted and a successful solution can be devised.

Living with Tourette Syndrome means making some accommodations, but it shouldn't mean becoming a recluse. There's a fine balancing act between doing what you want and living as normal a life as possible, and also appreciating that others have rights too.

CHAPTER 12

Managing Behavioral Problems

When you have a youngster with Tourette Syndrome, one of the hardest calls to make is in regard to behavioral problems: Is the problem an expression of the Tourette Syndrome or is he (or she) just acting up today?

Unfortunately, there is no clear-cut answer. The reason that there really is no definitive way to analyze behavior is due to the waxing and waning patterns of TS tics. Depression and mood swings may accompany TS, or they may reflect a child's lack of experience in handling disappointments and frustration. A new misbehavior may be naughtiness, but it also may be a new tic or compulsion that has suddenly appeared. It also may be an expression of your child's ADHD or OCD.

"My son stuck his tongue out at his teacher," a mother told me. "Naturally, she was shocked and sent him to the principal. Rather than saying it was a tic (albeit a new one), he was embarrassed and said nothing. When my husband and I found out, we punished him for being rude and disrespectful. It wasn't until later, when we noticed his sticking his tongue out while playing soccer with his friends, that we realized a new tic had appeared. We were angry at ourselves for not considering that possibility and furious with him for not telling us. We would have believed him. At least, I hope we would have."

Another parent confided that her son had punched holes in the walls of his bedroom. "We punished him by giving away the tickets we had gotten for him and his father to see a professional baseball game. Later, that night, he came to us and tearfully admitted that he had felt a compulsion to hit the wall. He hadn't been angry or frustrated, just compelled to smash his fist against the wall. When he had finally cracked the dry wall, he said he felt better. That's when we discovered that, in addition to Tourette Syndrome, our son suffered from obsessive-compulsive behavior. He smashed the wall once more. Then we bought him a punching bag and he beats the dickens out of it when he feels the need to hit. Usually, but not always, the substitute target satisfies that feeling for him.''

Parents need to become familiar with their child's personal patterns. Some youngsters give facial cues when they're about to lose control or can tell you when they feel an inner warning sensation. Often you can head trouble off at the pass by substituting another field of focus or by physically removing a youngster from a potentially difficult situation. If your child takes a swipe at the jigsaw puzzle the siblings are working on, take him in the next room and read to him or let him listen to music. Ask him to help you wash the car or run errands. If you sense that your daughter can't sit still any longer at the restaurant, take her outside or in the lobby and let her walk around. Activity often helps to disperse some of the tension that has built up.

Praise Often Please

Praise, offered sincerely, is one of the strongest inducements to improving behavior. I often use the acronym POP, which stands for ''Praise often please.''

We all like to be rewarded for working hard and doing the right thing. It's not just a kid thing. Businesses offer raises, bonuses, and other work-related incentive programs. The government and the military confer plaques and medals, and successful athletes collect trophies like the rest of us collect their playing cards.

Many of us have no trouble patting our dog or cat on the head, and offering praise when our pet shows desirable behavior, but we withhold the same ''warm fuzzies'' when it comes to our kids. Yet studies reveal that reinforcement of good behavior increases its frequency. Rather than focusing on your child's poor behavior, start praising and rewarding the actions you want to see more of, even if you feel silly at first.

Set up a specific reward and punishment system so your child knows what is expected and what the consequences are for failure to perform as desired.

- Start small. If you begin with too many rules, they'll be overwhelming. Your youngster will feel programmed for failure and give up trying to change.
- Be precise in describing what you consider to be acceptable and nonacceptable behavior. "Play nicely" or "Don't fight" are too vague. Try instead "Wait your turn" and "Don't throw the blocks," which are more specific.
- Discuss the plan with your child before implementing it so there is no misunderstanding.
- Offer a variety of rewards for short- and long-term good behavior, depending on your child's age. They can range from a sticker, toy, or books to a movie, trip to the zoo, or a personal telephone. Limit your use of food as rewards, especially sweets.
- Be consistent. Once you've described the punishments for infractions, you must carry them out.
- Remember that *discipline* is not synonymous with *punishment*. Everyone needs discipline, which means learning to act within certain guidelines or rules. Punishment is what happens when these rules are not followed. It's difficult enough having a child with TS. If you don't maintain proper discipline, you'll have a bratty youngster as well.
- Never use this type of program to bribe your child to stop ticcing. Use solely for altering or reducing accompanying behavior problems. It's especially effective when dealing with children who have ADHD along with TS.
- Don't ever underestimate the ingenuity of your offspring. When my children were little I developed a reward/ punishment system for them, giving each youngster ten poker chips for the week. Each child had his or her own color. For rule infractions, they were fined two chips; if they fulfilled their specific responsibilities, they received two

extra. At the end of each week, the poker chips could be traded in for "shopping spree with Mom," "one extra TV show," and other rewards.

On a particular day, one of my sons flew into a rage. He was fined two chips. He kept screaming and slugging, so he was fined two more, then two more. Finally, in complete frustration, he threw all of his chips at me. I then realized that there were more chips on the floor than he possibly could have saved up. He had taken his allowance, ridden his bike to the drugstore, and purchased extra boxes of poker chips in his color. It was hard keeping a straight face. I suggest using payment tokens that can't be counterfeited.

• Never underestimate the power of verbal praise in altering behavior. A "Well done" or "I'm so proud of you," a hug or pat on the back, or telling a friend on the phone of good behavior (when your child is in listening distance) works wonders.

How to Distinguish Tics from "Time-Out" Behavior

Youngsters, being only human, often will play one parent against the other, teacher against parent, or just use Tourette Syndrome for their own benefit.

The messages we give—verbally or through body language—are quickly received and internalized. If there are no behavioral boundaries—if everything is accepted because "my poor child has TS and can't help what he's doing"—then a youngster learns that anything goes and begins to take advantage of his disorder. Parents, teachers, and doctors may subconsciously encourage children to continue the role of "little sick kid." It will take a long time to change that image they have of themselves.

For example, spitting may be one of your child's tics and therefore has to be accepted as involuntary. If he or she can't substitute a more acceptable tic, however, the tic can be tempered by learning to turn away or by using a handkerchief so the spitting isn't at another person, on food or school papers.

A child with coprolalia finds it difficult to control the obscenities that erupt, often to everyone's shock and embarrassment. If your youngster has this type of tic, you must learn to acknowledge it and help suggest ways to substitute other words or mask what's being said, if possible. If you hear your child using swear words to attack a playmate, you need to ask, "Is this your tic or are you angry at your friend?" If it's the latter, you need to explain what's permissible and what isn't. Be firm about it. Kids need limits and want to know their boundaries. Well-meaning parents and teachers make things worse when they set none.

- *Encourage open communication.* Bite your tongue when you're about to become judgmental. Agree on a sign or signal, so words aren't necessary in public.
- *Develop a sense of trust.* Open communication should provide a comfort zone, so that if your child says the behavior is involuntary, you know it's true. Show how important trust is in a relationship through your own example.
- *Avoid stressful situations when your youngster is fatigued.* Just as a diabetic youngster must learn how stress affects his or her insulin requirements, your child must begin to take responsibility for his or her chronic condition. Practice stress reduction yourself.
- *Plan ahead so your child has "escape routes."* Eventually it will become second nature for your child to take a seat to the side in school (so that others won't see the tics) or sit by the door in the lunchroom in order to leave quickly to express the tics or keep from slugging someone.
- *Explain behavior difficulties to those in charge before they are displayed.* It helps when those in charge know what to expect so they can head off potential problems in advance.
- *Decide which rules are most important. Keep the list short.* Children with ADHD and TS become overwhelmed with too many rules. They often end up unable to follow any of them. Be sure your child knows the penalty for breaking a rule.
- *Help siblings understand why they're not permitted to display behavior that is acceptable for the youngster with TS.* Spend time one-on-one with each child to keep your lines of communication open.

- *Be consistent in both your reactions and punishment.* Youngsters need to know where the line is drawn. If the line wavers according to your mood or time of day, it's confusing. Use "time-out" as a way to take a child away from a situation in which he or she has misbehaved, not as a respite for you.
- *Balance the punishment with the offense.* It's easy when you're frustrated and exhausted from listening to your child's vocal tics to overreact when she misbehaves. "No TV for a month," you scream. Try to separate your own fatigue, guilt, and sense of helplessness from your response and deal as unemotionally with the offense as possible.
- *Make some time for yourself.* No one will give you personal time—you have to make it. Plan it into each day as though it is important. It is.

CHAPTER 13

Handling Siblings' Reactions

Siblings of a child with Tourette Syndrome often are the "shadow children." Parents get so caught up with what is happening with the TS youngster—from confusion over the symptoms, to seeking out and finally arriving at the diagnosis, to determining treatment and then constantly juggling side effects from the medications—that they often forget they have other kids who don't have TS.

Of course, as one mother interjected, "But my kids without TS *do* have obsessive-compulsive disorder and attention deficit disorder with hyperactivity, so everyone has something. We play no favorites here." She and many others I interviewed displayed one important skill vital to having a child with Tourette Syndrome: developing and maintaining a sense of humor.

Is It My Fault?

Children (as well as many adults) often tend to assume the responsibility when misfortune befalls a family member. Siblings may feel they caused their brother or sister to have TS, because they were angry at him or her and wished something bad would happen. They may have felt resentful over the attention the TS child received from the parents before the diagnosis and then guilty once they realize that something really *is* wrong.

Because it often takes months or even years between recognition of the first expression of symptoms and a confirmation of the diagnosis, chances are good that most parents have worried about and fussed over the child with Tourette Syndrome for a long time, vainly attempting in a myriad of ways to get him or her to stop the tics. It doesn't really matter if the attention has been positive or negative. As a matter of fact, many siblings admitted (without their parents being present) that they sometimes got into trouble too, just to get their parents to notice them, even if it meant being yelled at or punished.

Be aware that you may be reinforcing bad behavior in your other children without realizing it. Although it's hard for most of us to carve out any extra time in our hectic lives, it's important to try to spend some special time with each child, even if it's no more than ten or fifteen minutes. When my children were small, I utilized drive time for that. The kid was captive in the car and couldn't go anywhere. We turned off the radio and talked with no subject forbidden.

A quick trip to the cleaners once was accompanied by conversation concerning whether or not to try out for track, what English class to take next semester, and why guys you really like act the stupidest when you're around. There also was a small complaint, unobtrusively slipped in between the other chatter, about how unfair it was to always have to sit next to the sibling who sniffed constantly in the movies. "It makes me tic more," she said.

It was an enlightening statement and (thankfully) one that could easily be resolved. Without that one-on-one time she probably wouldn't have said anything until it had grown into a major problem. That conversation and others like it made running errands extra productive.

This time not only focuses your undivided attention but it also provides an opportunity to reassure your other children that they were not to blame for their sibling's having Tourette Syndrome. Nothing they said, wished, or did caused it; it was just bad genetic luck.

One-on-one time also allows your other children the opportunity to express how they feel—embarrassment from the TS sibling's tics, anger that they have to defend him or her from taunts from schoolmates, or concerns, such as whether they will develop Tourette Syndrome too. Make time to listen, be supportive, and be thankful that your children feel comfortable in sharing their true feelings with you.

Sometimes youngsters may be reluctant to express their emotions for fear you'll be angry or that it isn't loyal to feel resentful. If you suspect that to be the case, admit that sometimes you also feel relief in getting away from the constant tics, and that you also have a multitude of feelings, ranging from anger and frustration to sadness that your child has a chronic disorder. Describe the ways that you have learned to cope so your children understand that everybody has something to deal with in life.

A mother with four children, two of whom have TS with ADD and OCD, and two of whom have ADD and OCD respectively, said that coping with her children's disorders had made the entire family grow closer and taught them to be more understanding of the problems other people face. This thought was echoed by the majority of the parents and young people I interviewed. One young adult went so far as to say that he felt that those with Tourette Syndrome had "a special gift. They are capable of seeing other people when they are hurting and be sensitive to their pain. We understand other people's pain and their needs," he concluded.

You may discover that the TS child's younger siblings have some of the same guilty feelings as the older ones and need to be reassured as well. In addition, they may worry about catching TS. While you need to remind younger children that Tourette Syndrome is not a contagious disease, you should never promise that they won't develop it; they might.

Most younger children look up to the older ones in the family, trying to emulate them in every way. When the older child has TS, this hero worship often doesn't develop. A younger sibling may be disappointed and keenly feel the loss. Help your children to see past the TS and to accept one another as individuals. Highlight the specialness inherent in each of us.

Reactions from Siblings

Reactions from your other children to both the diagnosis and the disorder itself may vary widely. As with parents, some children may be relieved to learn that their sibling's strange behavior is something that cannot be controlled, that it is involuntary. It also has a name, so if they are teased by their peers, they now have a retort: "He can't help it. He has Tourette Syndrome and that's why he makes those movements and noises."

The more information you share with the siblings and the more they are included in early discussions with the physician and support groups, the less likely they are to feel like outsiders or that anything is being kept from them. You may think that your other children, whatever their ages, are too young to be burdened with all the problems inherent in Tourette Syndrome and its possibly concurrent disorders. But by attempting to protect them, you surround them with walls of ignorance. These shadow siblings grope their way outside the family circle, and because of their lack of knowledge, conjure up frightening scenes of what might be.

"I thought my brother was going to die," a twenty-four-year-old sibling confided in me. "My parents whispered about his condition behind closed doors. Nobody told me anything. I could have been more supportive when we were in junior high and high school if I'd only known what was going on. As it was, I alternated between feeling resentful of him and feeling guilty that I felt resentful! Sometimes I joined in the teasing because I didn't know why he did those things. I thought he was doing them on purpose."

Other siblings confessed that they never brought friends over to their house. "It was bad enough at school," said one. "My friends didn't need to hear the garbage that came out of my brother's mouth here at home too." Later, however, after giving a speech on Tourette Syndrome in her psychology class, this same young woman was surprised to have friends come up to her and say, "Oh, that must be what your brother has. Is that why he cusses and blinks all the time?" Education often does make people more understanding. Educate your own kids first, then encourage them to share their newfound knowledge with friends. You'll have to adjust explanations so they're appropriate to your children's ages. The TSA has brochures and videos such as "Stop It, I Can't" and "A Regular Kid, That's Me," especially written for youngsters.

Keep them—as well as members of your extended family—within the information circle. Each of you needs the emotional support from the others; that's what families do.

Tell the parents of your child's friends too, so they can explain it to their youngsters. Call the disorder by its real name, Tourette Syndrome, not a "habit." The word *habit* implies that a person can overcome something by exerting discipline and willpower. Your child can't turn the tics off by willing them away.

It's natural to want to shield your children from pain—physical or emotional. But it's easy to become overprotective when your child has TS. We don't want them to experience failure, embarrassment, or lack of acceptance. But all of those occurrences are part of life and are learning experiences on which to build coping mechanisms that will carry youngsters into and throughout adulthood. If children never face any of these obstacles, they won't know how to handle them when we're not around.

Listen carefully when your other children complain that you overprotect the sibling with TS. Kids usually have a sense of fair play. They may be revealing an important issue.

"He hit me and you just say, 'oh, it's his tic. Forget about it.' But it wasn't his tic. He really slugged me. I know the difference," one youngster wailed to his mother. Another complained, "You always excuse her for everything she does and then blame me instead. I *know* she's got TS, but she gets out of doing anything she doesn't want to do and gets to do anything she wants. Why don't you ever tell her 'no'?"

We probably limit saying "no" because we ache when any of our children are in pain. But by preventing our youngster with Tourette Syndrome from experiencing hurts and failures and learning from them, we're suggesting that he or she isn't very capable, that the other kids can cope with failure, but that our "fragile" TS child cannot. Before we know it, that youngster will give up trying, figuring that "Mom and Dad don't think I can handle this."

It's tempting to provide a safe haven where you can harbor and protect your child against stupid comments, hurtful taunts, stares by strangers, and embarrassment. Ironically, our love and support can sometimes be so overpowering that our unspoken message is, "You're safe here at home with us. *We* accept you; your peers may not." The child feels so comfortable and secure with us that he or she has no need for peers. The family fills that role. Unfortunately, all that does is prolong the inevitable, and when that young person does venture out, it is without the self-confidence and social skills that we, through misguided love, have prevented him or her from developing.

Siblings of children with chronic illness take their cues from the parents. If you and your spouse are fearful about allowing your youngster with TS to experience life—to attend school, make friends, join a club, play sports, fall in love, be rejected, and, yes, even to fail—then your other children will sense that the sibling with TS is vulnerable and needs protection. Rather than being understanding and supportive, they may become overprotective too and smother their brother or sister even as they try to envelop their sibling in a sheltering cocoon.

Coping with Tension and Stress

Living with someone with Tourette Syndrome can be extremely stressful. Youngsters don't want to stand out. Having a brother or sister who is different—who has TS—puts the spotlight on the sibling as well.

Some kids have the innate maturity to be able to shake it off. Most, however, are embarrassed and occasionally either join in with the teasing or become angry at the sibling for bringing unwanted attention to them both, despite understanding that the tics and embarrassing behavior are involuntary.

Rather than taking up for the child with TS and launching into a "How could you do this to your brother when you know he can't help it?" speech, focus instead on the feelings of your child without Tourette Syndrome. "I guess you must have felt very embarrassed." Rather than assigning blame or piling on guilt (chances are he feels rotten about his actions by now anyway), you have acknowledged his feelings, are sensitive to the situation, and may have some suggestions, which, of course, you do.

1. Encourage him to explain what Tourette Syndrome is to his friends, being sure to include that it is a neurological disorder (not emotional), and that the tics are involuntary.
2. Make sure that he is able to answer all of his friends' questions—which means that he needs to be fully informed too.
3. Urge him to develop and keep a sense of humor. Making light of a stressful situation can often defuse the tension.
4. Recommend that he spends some time away from the sibling with TS. Even if both youngsters are close in age, each needs to develop some friends of his own. Forcing the child with TS to always tag along causes resentment on the part of both children.
5. Arrange for him and each child to have a sanctuary—a room, closet, drawer, or desk—where personal papers and treasures are safe from prying eyes. Provide a padlock, if necessary. This is especially important if your youngster with TS also has ADHD and may break or damage a sibling's possessions.
6. Remind him that each child is special in his or her own way. Encourage him to do his best to develop his own talents and not to feel guilty that his sibling has TS. This message relieves pressure on your other children who may worry that their parents feel that they are trying to show up the youngster with TS when they succeed. The child with TS also has strengths and must be encouraged to develop those as well. Never compare your children's achievements, just praise them.

Support Groups for Siblings

Many communities offer special programming for siblings of youngsters with various disabilities. One such program is called Sibshop, which originated at Children's Hospital in Seattle in 1982. At this writing there are more than eighty Sibshop groups in the United States and more than twenty in Canada.

According to the director of the Sibling Support Project, Donald Meyer, Sibshop "seeks to provide brothers and sisters of children with special needs opportunities for peer support and education." The youngsters quickly learn that they are not alone in having a sibling with special needs. Through a relaxed and recreational setting, these youngsters share concerns as well as solutions common to all. Most of the sessions are four hours and also include fun activities such as cooking, juggling, and offbeat games.

CHAPTER 14

Reducing Stress

Coping with Tourette Syndrome and any of its concurrent problems can create considerable emotional stress on the entire family, especially when the TS symptoms are particularly severe. Unrelieved, this negative stress can trigger a number of physical and emotional disorders including digestive upsets, headaches, high blood pressure, skin problems, and depression. Constant stress can weaken your immune system, leaving you more vulnerable to infection, and respiratory and cardiac problems.

While stress is a normal part of life that we all must learn to handle, families dealing with Tourette Syndrome, ADHD, and OCD (or with any chronic disorder) especially must seek out and practice ways of coping with negative stress in order to keep themselves physically and emotionally healthy.

While other chapters in this section have dealt with specific actions families can take to handle the *physical* effects of TS on the family, this chapter highlights ways in which parents or a spouse can gain relief from the emotional pressures of having a family member with a chronic disorder that affects behavior.

During the course of researching this book, I interviewed many families having more than one child with Tourette Syndrome. Some of these children also had ADHD, some had TS with OCD, and some had all three disorders. I was struck by their "We can do it" attitude.

"I think it's made us closer as a family," said one mother of four children, two with TS, ADD, and OCD. "We've all had to become pretty creative sometimes in dealing with some of these problems. Having a strong religious faith has helped get me back on track when I waver. But,'' she admitted with a smile, "sometimes my husband and I have to get away a while just to keep us in balance.''

Running Away

The need for respite was voiced frequently by the majority of these families. Parents who juggle daily demands of work, child care, household chores, and perhaps care for elderly parents as well, may be bent to the breaking point as they deal with the constancy of behavioral problems, vocal tics, and the need to settle conflicts with school, siblings, peers, and extended family. When both parents are involved, there may be additional friction emanating from different parenting styles; when there is only a single parent, the burden of being responsible for everything may be overwhelming. Even the most loving spouse of someone with TS may also feel the occasional need to escape temporarily. Some time off, an approved running away, is required.

But how? How do you find a qualified baby sitter for an eight-year-old with verbal and motor tics who is also hyperactive and obsessed with taking the electrical plates off of the wall sockets, washing rocks in the bathtub, and chewing on batteries? Where do you find someone to stay with your ten-year-old who requires the delicate balancing of medication, punches holes in the walls, and spends hours washing his hands?

"I can't ask my in-laws to spell me,'' one mother complained. "They think I'm too hard on my son and will give in to him just to keep the peace. They don't seem to understand that discipline is vital for him. He *has* to have boundaries or he'll explode in four directions at once like a fire cracker. The rules help him to control his hyperactivity and compulsions, and even reduce the frequency of a few of his tics.''

While many parents do utilize help from the grandparents, others trade off with other parents they have met in either the local TS group or their area's Children and Adults with Attention Deficit Disorder (CH.A.D.D.) chapter. "We have too many kids for one family to handle,'' said a father, ''so we divide the kids up. The TS kids go with a family familiar with medication and behavioral problems and the other two go to their grandparents.''

One set of parents set up strict bedtimes for their children. "They don't have to be sleeping, but they do have to stay in their rooms," they said. "That way a sitter can come to the house and shouldn't have to deal with too many problems. We also give a little prize if they don't budge from their rooms while we're away. It's the only way we've found to go out for an occasional movie or dinner without worrying about what's happening at home.''

Some families utilize students from nearby medical or nursing schools as sitters. It offers firsthand experience in dealing with TS, ADD, and/or OCD to these future medical professionals and expands their awareness and knowledge of these disorders, a real service considering a recent study by CH.A.D.D., which revealed that most pediatricians received only two hours of training in attention deficit disorders while they were in medical school.

Never be reluctant to ask for help from friends, coworkers, relatives, and health-care professionals. It's vital to create a backup team that best suits the individual needs of your particular family. Don't play the martyr and feel that you're indispensable. You're not. Some time just for you, both individually and as a couple, should revitalize and help strengthen your marriage, which gives your kids a strong sense of support. They need to know that regardless of how bad their symptoms get, it won't break up the family.

Single parents must schedule some time off as well, without feeling guilty or apologetic for needing it. You're carrying a double load, which makes it even more important for you to line up a reserve team now. It will help your youngster feel less frantic if you ever are sick or have to be away on business and will make him or her less dependent on just you. This is especially important as your child gets closer to adolescence, a period in which most young people want to become more independent, draw away from parents, and identify with peers. Because children with Tourette Syndrome often need more parental intervention due to medication regulations and school support, helping them feel comfortable with a substitute parental figure may help bridge that difficult period.

There are other advantages in giving yourself some time away, even if it's only a few hours. It allows you an opportunity to consider discipline and other problem areas more objectively, away from the emotions of the moment; it permits pampering time, something we all need, whether it's shopping, getting a facial or a manicure, going fishing, or wandering through an art gallery or museum without worrying what your child is up to. A holiday from constant responsibility puts you in touch with your own needs, emotions, and strengths. You'll return home more rested, mentally healthier, and better able to handle stresses in your life.

Exercise

Exercise offers psychological support as well. Exercise is nature's form of tranquilizer as it triggers the production of chemicals that create a sense of relaxation and well-being. It also reduces the extreme fatigue of depression, a normal response when you're faced with the frustrations attendant with TS and its concurrent disorders. Even commercial dieting programs now acknowledge that exercise also helps to control weight by boosting the metabolism, which causes you to burn calories at a faster rate.

According to the experts, the best form of exercise is one that you enjoy. If plain old walking doesn't appeal to you, find something that does. Try biking—stationary or regular—stair climbing, hiking, swimming, skating, line dancing, running, tennis, racquet ball, or jumping rope. There's bound to be some form of exercise that pleases you. Don't be too quick to purchase exercise equipment like treadmills or cross-country ski machines, however. Rent first to see how you like using them.

Although many people prefer to exercise alone, making it their special time so they can let their mind wander and feel totally free from responsibility, some parents encourage their children to exercise with them. It offers special benefits for the child with TS:

1. It may help to reduce the severity or frequency of the tics.
2. It's a positive way to work off excess energies.

3. It gives your child the same benefits as it does you.
4. Exercise is a good way for your youngster to spend quality time with you.
5. It gives you both a common interest.

Whether you exercise alone or with your youngster, you'll soon discover that regular exercise improves self-esteem. You'll feel better, have improved muscle tone, be more relaxed and stronger emotionally, ready to handle whatever difficulties Tourette Syndrome, ADD, or OCD sends your way.

(NOTE: Always get a physical checkup from your physician before starting any exercise program.)

Relaxation Techniques

I asked a single mother with three children with Tourette Syndrome if she ever used meditation or relaxation techniques to help reduce the stress present in her daily life. She shook her head. "No, I just pray a lot."

Actually, prayers can be a form of relaxation. They take you away from the tension of your daily life. Familiar prayers, recited by rote, are similar to the mantra used by those who practice yoga or self-hypnosis. Both allow you to narrow your focus, shutting out all other stimuli.

I use progressive relaxation, just one of many relaxation techniques, to help me unwind. Despite some of the books that try to make it sound complicated and somewhat mysterious, it's really easy to learn. The theory behind it is fairly simple: If you're relaxed, you can't be tense. Picture the toddler who runs around in the park, then zonks out on your shoulder on the way home.

Get comfortable in a chair, recliner, or on the bed. Then inventory your body, identifying any tension present. Allow it to dissipate while you visualize some scene that is soothing to you. It's different for everybody. For some, it may be floating gently in an air balloon or sunning on a sandy beach. For my niece, it's jumping out of an airplane—with a parachute on, of course. For me, it is sitting on an old-fashioned swing and swaying back and forth on a hill overlooking a harbor filled with sailboats bobbing up and down on their anchor lines.

Concentrate on your breathing and focus on your personal place. Tell your body to relax, beginning with your forehead, cheeks, and chin, and so on down to your toes, letting the tension fade out the end of your toes. Tell each part of yourself to relax.

"I try," you may complain, "but everything I have to do pops into my head and makes me tense again."

That's a natural occurrence and why you need to practice the technique. Don't fight the thoughts that enter your mind; rather let them float away like bits of fluffy clouds in the sky. When they try to reattach themselves, just think "relax" or "peace," "love," or whatever word you choose, and drift like a kite blown by a gentle breeze in the sky. Sail to your private place in your mind. It's impossible to think two thoughts at once. If you're thinking "relax," you can't think "car pool."

There are many different relaxation techniques to sample. You'll find numerous books describing them in your library or bookstore. Probably the best known on relaxation is *The Relaxation Response* by Herbert Benson, M.D. There also are many audiotapes available to help you relax.

"The idea," a relaxation expert told me, "is not to withdraw from the world, but to be equipped to handle stressful situations by being able to relax and release the tension you feel."

After practicing whatever technique you choose—experts suggest about twenty minutes a day—you'll soon find that you can release tension easily as you wait for a red light to change, while you're at home with the kids or at work trying to stay ahead of a deadline. Closing your eyes even briefly, as you concentrate on your deep breathing and allow the tension to float away, will help you feel more in control. But in order to achieve this, you need to make time for relaxation.

While you may think that you don't have time to do one more thing, please reconsider. If you don't take care of yourself first, you'll be in no shape to help others. That's why the instructions on airplanes concerning the use of oxygen always emphasize putting your own mask on first.

Equally important, our kids mimic what they see. When they notice you using relaxation to control your tension level, they may become interested in learning a technique that works for them as well. It may be different from the one you've selected. Encourage them to keep trying until they find a good fit.

Experts suggest that children with TS actually tic less when they utilize relaxation techniques to minimize stress and fatigue. Some youngsters bring a recorder and relaxation tape to school so they can listen to it when they feel particularly "ticcy." Many schools offer relaxation and stress training for all their students. Relaxation is a life skill, one all children should learn, regardless if they have Tourette Syndrome or not.

Touch Therapy

If you're not a toucher and don't like to be touched, this section may not be for you. If you're lukewarm, read on. This may start your family on a whole new way of communicating. I happen to be a toucher and feel comfortable saying to my husband or any of my kids, "I need a hug." According to Sherry Suib Cohen, coauthor of *The Magic of Touching,* "You can't give a touch without getting one right back. You can talk, listen, smell, see, and taste alone, but touch is a reciprocal act."

Our language is filled with references to the act of touching. "You really touched me," "Give me a hand," and even the telephone commercial, "Reach out and touch someone," all underscore the importance of touching. Medical science has proven that premature babies and geriatric patients alike fare better when they are tactually stimulated. The physical and emotional healing that comes from the "laying on of hands" is no myth.

"Sometimes, when my child's tics seem to be on fast forward, I just hug him," one mother said. "I can feel the tension draining out of him as the tics subside." Other parents described rubbing their children's neck, back, or just rocking them and watching the hyperactivity slow down. (Some children, however, don't like to be cuddled or held. Respect their preference.)

These soothing touches are also important for other members of the family. Everyone should be encouraged to ask for a hug or cuddle when they are needed. Don't expect your loved ones to be mind readers. Asking to be held never minimizes its effects.

Massage

Massage is a therapeutic form of touching that has been used for centuries to improve circulation and reduce stress. While there are a variety of styles—Swedish, sports, Shiatsu—all involve pressure, kneading, or stroking. You may need to experiment to determine which form of massage you prefer.

People also differ in their preference in background music while having a massage. Some prefer silence—no music, no conversation from the massage therapist. Don't hesitate to state your desire. After all, you're the client.

Many spas, beauty shops, hotels, and health clubs offer the services of a massage therapist. You can also find qualified people by contacting rehabilitation centers, orthopedists, or the physical education department of a college or university. Be sure to check references, especially if the massage therapist is coming to your home. Many states require licensing. If yours is one of them, ask to see the person's credentials.

Massage not only helps to work out kinks in your neck and back, but it also helps dissolve tension in the rest of your body, improves circulation, and reduces overall stress.

Minimassage—the hand-kneading from a manicurist, scalp-rubbing from the barber, a facial or pedicure—are just other forms of informal touching that can ease stress and make you healthier both emotionally and physically. If nothing else, all these forms of touching force you to take some time off for yourself and remind you that your needs are important too.

Music

Studies have shown that soothing music can lower respiration, blood pressure, and pulse rate even for patients under anesthesia.

Many surgeons now routinely ask their patients what type of music they prefer before performing an operation.

The same relaxing effects of music can help you to reduce your stress level. Practice progressive relaxation while listening to your favorite calming music. Experiment with New Age or symphonic works to see if you find them effective. Instrumental renditions of old favorites can work as well, providing you don't find yourself mentally singing along. Experts suggest that the beat of the music should be close to that of your resting heartbeat—about sixty-five to eighty minutes.

Diaries

Many of us remember a diary as the imitation leather book with a lock and key that we received for Christmas or Chanukah when we were young. We faithfully made entries for the first few weeks in January, scribbled notes sporadically in February, and lost it in the back of the closet or under the bed by March.

The type of diary to help reduce stress is not as fancy. It has no prenumbered months and dates. There's no use adding more tension to your life by feeling you've nothing to say on specific days. Instead, think of this diary as a recording device to set down your thoughts and emotions when you need to express them.

Some people prefer the composition bound-book variety; some the spiral notebook; still others rely on the computer. Use whatever seems comfortable. Some weeks you may write nothing at all. At times, you may have more than one entry per day. The important thing is to express yourself without mentally editing what you write in your journal.

I can personally vouch for the stress-reducing effectiveness of having a journal. I kept a diary when I first learned that I had breast cancer, writing down my deepest feelings, some of which I was not yet ready to share with anyone, including my husband. I scribbled down my worst fears, my most "unworthy" thoughts, my objective observations, and even the things that made me laugh. Yes, there *were* things that tickled my funny bone, even then.

It was almost fifteen years before I reread what I had written.

I wept for the depth of emotion I found there, but remembered that the act of writing those words and expressing my feelings had helped to keep me going while I was preparing for surgery and undergoing follow-up treatment.

Encourage your children—the child with TS and siblings too—to keep journals of their thoughts as well. It might be difficult for the one with TS, especially if there are learning difficulties, severe motor tics, and/or ADHD, but many young people have reported that the struggle was well worth the effort, because "telling" their journal how they felt helped to reduce some of their stress.

Jason Valencia, a young man with Tourette Syndrome, permitted two of the poems he had written to be included in the Illinois TSA newsletter. One of the poems was written when Jason was ten years old, the second, when he was seventeen. He graciously has permitted me to include them in this book.

TOURETTE KIDS
by Jason Valencia (age ten in 1986)

Sometimes we are happy
Sometimes we are sad.
Sometimes we get teased
Sometimes we get mad.

Although we seem different
when tics appear each day,
remember this disease chose us
and not the other way.

So if we jerk or yell or swear
please try not to forget
it isn't us doing it
but a disease called Tourette.

DIFFERENCES
by Jason Valencia (age seventeen in 1993)

Who are you to judge
because I'm not the same as you?
Some actions and some words I say,
I do not voluntarily do.

Who are you to make me cry
because you think odd of what you see?
Have you never given a second thought
to take a deeper look at me?

If you look beyond my physical traits
and see the person inside,
You'll see how tough my struggle is
fighting something I'm not able to hide.

Maybe I spit, maybe I swear,
or constantly tap my hand.
How do I explain these things to you,
when I, myself, don't understand?

Yes, it hurts me deep inside
when I hear the taunting words you say.
And you, my friend, may need me near
when *you* get judged one day.

Understand that I'm not crazy,
I'm not trying to make you mad.
Understand I have unique problems,
that I'll probably always have.

I don't expect you to treat me
differently, nor cut me lots of slack.
The only thing I ask of you is,
please, don't turn your back.

Such is the power of the pen. Encourage your children to develop their writing skills not only to express how they feel today but to carry their thoughts into their adult years as well. Then practice what you preach.

Hobbies

Hobbies are another way to reduce your stress level. What they are varies tremendously and what relaxes you may be stressful for me, either because I find it terrifying or boring. If you think you don't have time for a hobby, think again. You can't afford not to.

A hobby may be something you do alone, such as gardening, writing poetry, sewing, reading, playing an instrument, stamp collecting, or fishing. For some, exercise may be their hobby. Others may find that their hobby, which began as a solo pursuit, has led them to join with others sharing a similar interest.

It's especially important for parents with children who have TS or any chronic disorder to develop some type of a hobby as it not only serves as a stress-reducing momentary escape but it also gives you something else to think and talk about. Living with a chronic disorder in your family has an insidious effect on your thinking and conversation. One day you suddenly realize that the disorder is dominating your life, mind, and soul. You have no thought that doesn't revolve around it; your every conversation is peppered with references to it. "It" has won.

"No wonder I don't have any friends left," one woman mused. "My only acquaintances are other parents whose kids have Tourette Syndrome. I've been obsessing about my daughter's TS without being aware of it." As many parents of children with TS suffer from OCD themselves, it's easy for this to happen. Guard against it. Sharing a hobby with people outside your TS circle will help you to enjoy a fuller and less stressful life.

Consider becoming involved in one activity or organization that is not TS related. While most of us throw our time and energies into working with the TS, OCD, and ADD support groups because that *is* the main focus of our lives and we deal with it every day of our lives, it's important to have one outside activity as well—teaching Sunday School, having a Cub Scout troop, learning sign language, or being a docent at a museum or art gallery. It widens your circle of friendships, allows you to meet new people (whom you also can educate about TS), and gives you an extra time-out for yourself to reduce your stress so you're better able to focus on your child's needs when you return home.

Laugh and Cry

Tears of joy and sadness are a healthy expression of emotion and one that you should allow. The physical act of laughing releases chemicals in the brain called *endorphins* into the bloodstream, creating a sense of relaxation and well-being. Hearty laughter, the kind we call belly laughter, causes you to breathe in deeply, bringing more oxygen into your lungs.

In *Anatomy of an Illness,* a book by the late Norman Cousins, he described how he had used the power of laughter to help cure him of a painful and crippling disease. While laughter won't make Tourette Syndrome go away, a sense of humor can help the entire family over many rough spots—even embarrassment from some of the tics. It's good for young people to learn early that it's okay to laugh at yourself, that life doesn't always have to be real and earnest. Sometimes it can just be downright ridiculous.

Bring laughter into your family by getting together with friends who love laughter, renting comedy videotapes and audiotapes, cutting cartoons out of the newspaper and taping them to the refrigerator, getting cartoon and joke books from the library or bookstore, and retelling humorous family stories.

Leonard Felder, Ph.D., coauthor of *When a Loved One Is Ill,* suggests using humor to defuse the stress of feeling guilty about not doing more to ease the way for our chronically ill child. "Imagine just for fun that the *Guinness Book of World Records* has asked you to be a finalist for a new category—'The caregiving family member who has the most guilt feelings in a single month.'" By carrying this thought to the absurd, Felder says we can see the humor of our efforts in trying to be perfect. He concludes, "I urge anyone who frequently feels self-critical to begin using a sense of humor and a sense of perspective to snap out of guilt whenever it begins to dominate your thoughts. We all need to laugh at ourselves every so often, especially when we are acting like the world's champion of guilt."

Similarly, we need to give ourselves permission to cry. If you have trouble letting yourself cry, read a sad book and let the tears flow; buy a ticket for a tear-jerker movie; listen to poetry or music and give in to your emotions. You'll find that those salty tears usually wash away your stress and sadness, and that you really *do* feel better after a good cry.

Counseling

If none of these methods for reducing stress seem to help, if you find yourself always fatigued, crying without a reason, unable to sleep or make decisions, you may be suffering from depression.

There's no need to suffer in secret, be embarrassed, or consider it a weakness. Don't wait longer than a few weeks, chiding yourself to "snap out of it." Depression is a real condition, but there is treatment for it. Get help from your physician, minister, priest or rabbi, a psychologist, psychiatrist, trained social worker, or other health-care professional.

Part IV

SCHOOL ISSUES

CHAPTER 15

Educating the Educators

School—a child's work. The cliche almost sounds lyrical, but often there's no music, only discord for a youngster with Tourette Syndrome. The uncontrollable verbal and motor symptoms create the unthinkable in a child's world: they make him different from the others.

According to Dr. Roger Kurlan of the Department of Neurology at the University of Rochester School of Medicine and Dentistry in Rochester, New York, "schooling probably represents the most significant focus of clinical management for children with TS. A survey of 200 child and adolescent cases of TS found that 30 percent of the population experienced learning problems." Numerous studies revealed that many of these youngsters had weaknesses in reading skills including oral reading and reading comprehension, writing skills and mechanics such as spelling and punctuation, and mathematics.

Fortunately, knowledge, caring, cooperation, and patience by both parents and teachers can ease the way and often help to initiate real learning for these youngsters and understanding by the child's peers and other school personnel. The key word is *knowledge*. To a teacher with no knowledge of TS, a child with the disorder is merely a disruptive element in the classroom, someone who clowns around, trying to attract attention and disturb the other students by impulsive behavior, inappropriate words and sounds, and who never seems to follow instructions. The noises destroy classroom discipline and the physical gyrations—jerking an arm out while holding a pencil or scissors or kicking—sometimes are potentially dangerous to the other children.

A teacher (and other school personnel such as nurses, guidance counselors, administrators, and coaches) who understands the condition, however, will be able to help the youngster with TS cope with the psychosocial problems associated with the disorder as well as devise solutions to make learning more productive.

In addition, it is often the classroom teacher who is the first to notice the tics and to suggest to the parents that the child may have Tourette Syndrome. According to Judy Wertheim, educator and author, "By merely being knowledgeable and informed on the subject and sharing their knowledge with their colleagues, teachers are in an excellent position to save many lives, not from death because Tourette Syndrome is not fatal, but from years of torment and embarrassment, and from the ultimate destruction of all self-esteem and motivation which so often leads to a wasted life." As 80 percent of all TS cases come to their physician self-diagnosed from reading an article, seeing a television program, or hearing about the disorder from a layperson, this role of the classroom teacher cannot be minimized.

Do Your Homework First

Every profession has its own special language that everyone in the field understands, but that leaves most outsiders confused. The education professions' dialect makes it extremely difficult for parents trying to access the system in order to help their children. Educators often speak in acronyms, usually without explaining what they mean: IEP (individualized education plan), LD (learning disabled), SED (socially or emotionally disturbed), LRE (least restrictive environment). Eventually, of course, we'll rattle off "IEP" and "on task" like pros, but during that perplexing learning curve period we worry that our kid's teachers and the school administration may think that *we* have learning problems as well because we don't seem to understand what they're telling us. We feel frustrated, angry, and helpless; the educators are puzzled as to why we don't understand "plain English."

In addition, it's easy to feel as though you're a foreigner within the school atmosphere itself. Like hospitals, schools are a world unto themselves. You don't know what the constant bells mean or where you're supposed to go, even as you dodge to keep from being trampled by hordes of students. But, if you're going to be effective in your child's school, you need to be extremely well prepared and informed *before* you call for that first appointment.

Preparing for the New School Year

For most parents, preparing for a new school year means shopping for whatever shoes and lunch boxes are "in" this season and buying pencils and notebooks. For the parents of a child with TS along with ADHD and/or OCD, however, it also means new teachers and the need for educating them about TS and the concurrent disorders along with the side effects of your child's medications.

• *Make it a team effort.* Most teachers want to help their students to do their very best in the classroom both educationally and socially. That's why they're teachers.

Make an appointment to talk to your child's teacher *before* the first day of class. If your youngster has more than one teacher, ask for a conference with them all. While it may seem simpler to just wait to talk to the teacher the first day of class, don't. Teachers are busy then, greeting their students, maintaining discipline, and setting the daily routine. Trying to focus on what you're saying at that hectic time will be difficult. By setting up a formal meeting beforehand, during the two or three preplanning days, before the children come back to class, you set the tone for the importance of what you have to say. You also show the teacher that you value him or her as a professional.

• *Have handouts available.* The Tourette Syndrome Association has materials available that are especially written for and by teachers, school nurses, and others in the administration. In addition to these excellent booklets, prepare a one-sheet list of your child's particular needs, citing both the problem as well as successful solutions from the past. Note such things as "Miss Johnson allowed Dan to go to the nurse's office when he felt the vocal tics were getting out of hand," or "As Emily's medication makes her more fatigued after lunch, her teacher at the previous school gave her tests and other stressful work before she ate."

• *Encourage the teacher to devise an emergency code.* Suggest to your child's teacher that a code be set up in advance, so your youngster can quickly be excused when the tics become overpowering and/or potentially out of hand. Most students can keep the tics in check for a short period, but eventually they have to be expressed. As one nine-year-old said, "It's like a sneeze that builds up. If I force it back, I have to keep thinking it down or it pops out. Eventually it's going to anyway." It takes a great deal of mental energy for a youngster to suppress these tics, energy that is drained from focusing on the school work at hand. The youngster usually knows when he can't be contained anymore. It prevents breakdown of classroom discipline if the child can come to the teacher's desk and say "Nurse's office" or "Butterfly," whatever the two have agreed upon, rather than just bolting from the room.

• *Be open and honest.* Your child is with the teacher most of the day, so you need to be perfectly frank. What situations make the tics worse? What, if anything, eases them? Are all kinds of physical activity all right or do some make your youngster more hyperactive? Does your child sometimes use TS as an excuse to get out of disagreeable tasks? What type of discipline works best? What is least effective?

• *Give the teacher permission to talk to the class* if *your child gives permission.* By making your child's teacher aware of the facts about TS and allowing him or her to discuss it with your child's classmates (when your child is not there), you empower the teacher to discount myths and allay any fears the other youngsters may have—that it may be catching, that your child's crazy, or may die from it. The more matter-of-fact the teacher is, the more understanding your child's classmates will be.

It's doubtful that your child is the only one with special problems. One year, in one of my children's classrooms, there was one youngster who was hearing impaired, another with hemophilia, and another with epilepsy. My child had Tourette Syndrome. That year, along with history, spelling, and math, the children learned a great deal about tolerance and focusing on each other's strong points, thanks to a caring teacher who understood each child's problems and special needs.

Older children often want to tell their classmates themselves. Many use their Tourette Syndrome, ADHD, or OCD as topics for term papers and speeches and usually find the other students fascinated, and more importantly understanding.

• *Write down the names and dosage of all medications your child takes as well as their possible side effects.* Do *not* refer to any pill as "the little yellow pill" or "the round white pill."

Most schools have an emergency medical card for each student. Be sure the names and dosage of all the medications your child takes are written down and spelled correctly. Add a description of each pill. Teachers do not dispense medicine; if medication needs to be taken during school hours, your child will have to go to the clinic or nurse's office. But if you've verified what pill and dosage is needed and when, there should be no problems. Check with your particular school.

By letting the teacher know what your child is taking along with the possible side effects, you have a valuable ally in helping to titrate the medication so the youngster has a reduction of the symptoms, but can still maintain normal function. Children perform differently at school than they do at home.

• *Smile.* You may be frustrated with what happened in last year's class or school, but this is a new year. You need the teacher's cooperation. Don't barge in with an adversarial attitude. Assume that this teacher wants to understand, cooperate, and help. You both can accomplish wonders by working in a united manner.

You may find that the teacher seems resentful and unwilling to cooperate with your suggestions. Stay objective. It's difficult because we feel very emotional when trying to get help for our kids. Consider the situation from the teacher's viewpoint.

"You may have developed a negative reputation," said one teacher. "Teachers, being human, talk in the lunchroom. It's one thing to discuss things with your child's classroom teacher, another to demand. Yours is just one of thirty or more children that this teacher—who also may have personal concerns totally unrelated to teaching—needs to give special attention to. Sharing information that can help the teacher is vital, but know when to back off. Don't overwhelm. Many parents are still angry, still mourning over their child. It's understandable, but yelling at your child's teacher won't change anything.''

• *Volunteer to help if your child isn't self-conscious.* I doubt that there's a teacher alive who would refuse an extra set of hands. There's always homework to correct, paperwork to be completed, tutoring, and numerous other time-consuming tasks. By volunteering for some of the work load, you show the teacher you understand what you're asking, and allow the teacher more time to work with your child.

• *Be diplomatic.* Although their purpose is to educate young people, schools are bureaucratic by nature. There is a definite hierarchy and you must quickly master it and work within its pecking order. Going over someone's head usually antagonizes that individual and makes it difficult for the person's superior to make decisions without creating utter chaos.

To a noneducator, some rules may not make sense; remember that they do, or at least seem to, for those in the profession. You will not change the system, but you *can* make it work for you by strengthening your communication skills (listening as well as speaking), not losing your temper, and remembering that your child's problems, although of vital importance to you and your youngster, are just one of many action items a particular teacher or school must handle each day.

• *Suggest to your child's teachers that as you both have the youngster's well-being at heart, you know they'll want to know what's been effective in the past.* It's an offer teachers can't refuse. Provide materials made available by the TSA.

• *If you disagree, be tactful.* Your mother was right: you catch more flies with honey than vinegar. Calling the teacher, principal, or other administrator ''rigid'' or ''stubborn'' may, in fact, be an accurate assessment, but it won't help your child. Try to understand why the school personnel is resisting and work within that framework to make it easy for them to adapt. If you present solutions rather than accusations, you'll usually find a climate of compromise. Just because "we've never done it that way," doesn't mean it can't be done. Choose your words as carefully as you do your child's medical treatment. Both can work wonders.

• *Keep your list of suggestions and requests brief.* Write them down so there's no misunderstanding. Phrase your proposals with the editorial "we," such as, "Why don't we try letting him tape his book report?" rather than, "Why don't you . . ."

• *Don't be defensive.* Although none of us likes to hear our child criticized, it *is* possible that our kid occasionally is to blame for misbehavior. Although a youngster with TS (and, possibly, OCD and ADHD) has a lot to handle, so does the teacher. It must be a team effort with both sides working together. For real success in the classroom, it cannot be a "them and us" situation. Be angry at the disorder, not at the teacher who is trying to deal with it in the classroom. Keep your communication free from fault-finding.

• *Organize an in-service training for the entire school.* Without it, you may have educated your child's third-grade teacher, but the following year, you'll have to start all over with the fourth-grade instructor. Also, as teachers are not the only adults coming into daily contact with your youngster, it's extremely important for others at school—the bus driver, lunchroom workers, library staff, and coaches—to understand what Tourette Syndrome is (and isn't), how the symptoms may vary, what discipline works best, how medication affects learning and behavior, and so on. If there is no one in your area whom you feel is qualified to present a factual in-service program, contact the TSA for assistance. Don't perpetuate any myths or yesterday's (now outdated) facts.

• *Two parents mean double clout.* As sexist as it sounds, schools are used to dealing with mothers. We've usually been the home-room mother, the chaperone on the field trip, the one who furnishes the cupcakes on birthdays or Halloween, and the PTA president. Teachers and the school administration are accustomed to mothers complaining about some unfair treatment their kid received. Even now, in the politically correct nineties, despite the fact that Mom may be the top executive in the bank or one of the partners in the law firm, she usually carries no extra status at her child's school.

When *both* parents come for a consultation, however, the administration sits up. "This must be important. Dad's here." As one educator said, "Schools respect seeing both parents." Then she hesitated. "But it's rare to see both."

A father's presence speaks volumes, showing (1) the family is united behind their youngster, (2) the parents are supportive and desirous of working with the school, and (3) the parents consider their child's well-being and success at school a top priority.

This double teaming is especially important for us as parents. When we come to a school conference, we're usually emotional. If your child has just been diagnosed, you're probably somewhat in shock as well. It's hard to focus on all that's been said. Sometimes we miss or misunderstand things. As we have our own agenda, we're often so busy talking that we forget to listen. That's where another set of ears comes in handy. Tape those sessions, not to prove anything later, but to play the tape back at leisure when you're more composed.

The word *parents* doesn't always mean the biological mother and father. It could be a custodial parent and stepparent, custodial grandparents, even one parent and the significant other. Family groupings vary tremendously in their composition today. It's impossible to list all possible combinations.

It can be very important for a significant other to attend these meetings to gain an understanding of what the child's parent is handling both physically and emotionally. It also tells a youngster who may still be feeling resentful of the parent's companion, "I care enough about you to learn how I can help too."

Addressing Special Needs in the Classroom

As with any other child with a chronic illness, children with TS have a variety of special needs, each as unique as the child.

About 50 percent of children with TS have minor problems that can be easily solved, while the remainder may require more specialized programs. One child may only need untimed testing or a place to go for time-out in order to do well in school, while another may need continual special help with reading, mathematics, and writing. Fortunately, for most children with TS, the educational difficulties tend to decrease once they are in their later teen years. Whatever aid is required, it must be given, as by federal law Tourette Syndrome is classified as a handicapping condition.

Although every school system has special teachers for learning-disabled children, most of these children also are mainstreamed for part of the day into classrooms with teachers who are not properly trained to help them. It is frustrating for the child, for the parents, and for the conscientious teacher who wants to help, but doesn't even understand the total problem, let alone the solution. According to Jacqueline Favish, M.Ed., a special education teacher and author, "Inclusion [the newer term for mainstreaming] is appropriate when it's appropriate. Sometimes it isn't."

"When I taught special education," Favish said, "there were two of us in the classroom, both of whom had masters degrees. We also had an aide and usually a student intern as well. That was for eight to twelve kids. If I, with all of my specialized training, sometimes had trouble knowing how to find a solution to some of the horrendous problems these kids face, what do you expect a 'regular' teacher with thirty kids to do?"

Who can help? Until the education departments of our universities wake up to the fact that *every* teacher, coach, and potential administrator needs to learn about TS, ADD, hyperactivity, OCD, and other problems affecting learning and classroom behavior, it must be the parent who fills that role.

In-service training, in which a particular school requests professional help for a specific "exception," solves part of the problem, but unless the nurse, social worker, or psychologist who is brought in is up-to-date on the latest data and fully comprehends all the subtleties involved with TS, he or she may be passing along misinformation. Parents of children with TS should always attend the in-service in order to hear what is being said and to personalize the symptoms and needs of their specific child. (NOTE: There are youngsters with TS who have conducted the in-service training at their schools).

Be sure that your school also has video and written materials made available by the Tourette Syndrome Association. A number of them are specifically written for the classroom teacher, school nurse, and school psychologist and deal with problems both in the classroom and with homework, ways to bolster a child's self-image at school, the importance of athletics and other self-esteem-building activities, social and interpersonal issues, school phobia, and how to cope with the symptoms in a classroom situation.

Some of these youngsters are under a tremendous burden in the school setting. One of the most vivid examples of how hard it can be for a child to cope with TS, OCD, and ADD was demonstrated recently at a workshop given by special education professional Susan Conners. She is a full-time French teacher and also has Tourette Syndrome.

"Most educators don't understand how much tics interfere with a student's ability to succeed in the classroom," she said. "I'm going to show you. Your assignment," she announced to the workshop attendees—teachers, parents, physicians, and me— "is to write the words to 'The Star Spangled Banner' in three minutes." As we picked up our pencils to begin, she waved her hand. "Wait. You haven't heard all of the instructions. You're a very impulsive group." She told us to begin to shake our heads. "That's your TS tic," she said. "Now, because you also have OCD, you have a finger and erasing compulsion. Every third word you must erase and rewrite. When I clap my hands, you must jab your finger on the desk three times. Begin—and you now have just two minutes and fifty-five seconds."

We picked up our pencils and began. She continued to talk, move books around, and clap her hands. I looked up and frowned. "Oh, I see you have an attention deficit as well," she said. There was scattered laughter. Everyone struggled to complete the assignment. Ms. Conners kept counting down on our allotted time. The workshop participants on each side of me slammed their pencils down in disgust, muttering "I lost my train of thought."

"Time's up," Conners said. No one had finished the assignment. I, along with others, had torn holes in my paper erasing it too hard. Some had completely forgotten the words to "The Star Spangled Banner" and were staring into space. Our actions had spoken far louder than words. It was a most vivid experience for us all.

Tips for Teachers

A number of internationally known special education teachers and psychologists, including Susan Conners, Jacqueline Favish, M.Ed., Harvey C. Parker, Ph.D., and Ramona Fisher-Collins, M.Ed., have determined and tested specific accommodations to help youngsters with Tourette Syndrome, attention deficit disorder, and obsessive-compulsive disorder experience success in the classroom.[1]

INATTENTION

Use side-front seating.
It's natural for teachers to seat children who are inattentive in the center front row, "where I can keep an eye on you." That's one of the worst places for children with Tourette Syndrome to sit because they know that everyone behind them can see their tics. They try harder to withhold the tics, which creates even more stress and ultimately makes the tics even worse.

Use support seating.
Seat the youngster in a section with strong role models surrounding his or her desk. If the neighboring students are attentive, it may serve as a reminder. Children are natural mimics.

---

[1] Reprinted by permission of the Tourette Syndrome Association, Inc., and by Harvey C. Parker, Ph.D., *A.D.D. WareHouse*, 300 NW Seventieth Avenue, Suite 102, Plantation, FL 33317.

Block distracting sounds.

If the student has ADD as well as TS, he or she may be distracted by classmates coughing, moving around in their seats, or sharpening pencils. Allow that child to wear headphones to listen to audiotapes of "white sounds" (the surf, rainfall, or breeze) or gentle instrumental music. These sounds may be distracting to some youngsters, but it's worth a try.

Establish listening cues.

Rather than singling out the child with TS and reminding him or her to stay on task, establish a hand cue—touching your nose or pulling your ear—to silently remind.

Simplify assignments.

Break all long-range assignments and instructions into smaller components. Have the child with TS do ten problems rather than twenty; turn in a two-page composition rather than eight pages. Supplement oral instructions with a one-page written summary. As with all of us, it's easy to procrastinate when you can't see the light at the end of the tunnel.

Verify written homework assignments.

Encourage the student to write down each homework assignment as it's given, then sign the sheet before the youngster leaves school. That helps parents to know that the work being done is actually what was assigned for homework. Some children prefer to tape record the homework assignment. You also can print it out each day and hand it to the youngster as he or she leaves class.

Allow extra time.

By allowing the child with TS extra time to complete a test or in-class assignment, you help him or her compensate for the time lost due to distractions, tics, and other difficulties. If other students complain about unfair advantage, remind them that everyone is different and that it has nothing to do with them.

Become aware of medication side effects.

The medications used to treat Tourette Syndrome as well as its concurrent disorders work because they change the chemical balance within the brain. Haloperidol (Haldol) is often effective in reducing the tics, but may cause side effects that you as a classroom teacher may notice before the child's parents.

Haldol, as well as pimozide (Orap), another drug used to treat TS, may interfere with a child's cognitive processes, and especially the short-term memory. What you may consider inattention and daydreaming could actually be the effect of these medications. Both Haldol and Orap also may make a youngster tired and appear drowsy or irritable. Another side effect of both medications is depression, which also causes a child to appear tired and inattentive. Many children actually may fall asleep in class, much to their embarrassment. Parents need to know of these reactions in order to report them to their child's physicians. Often it takes a great deal of experimentation until these medications are properly titrated, balancing tic reduction and side effects of the medications to everyone's satisfaction. Teachers must have information (from the parents or school nurse) concerning the effects of these medications in order to become informed observers.

ACADEMIC SKILLS

Obviously, inattention creates weakened academic skills. But that alone isn't the culprit. Equally at fault are the vast array of symptoms with which these youngsters must cope. As illustrated in the workshop exercise led by Susan Conners, it is also physically difficult for a child with TS to stay up with peers in the academic sphere. Effects of tics and medications make it exhausting to stay alert, focused, and on task. Yet a creative and understanding classroom teacher can introduce specific accommodations to compensate for some of these problems.

Devise reading aids.

One of my children had difficulty reading because he had a head tic. Every time his head jerked, he lost his place in the book.

Finally, we cut a rectangle out of a piece of cardboard. The rectangle covered the page in the book, leaving only the line he was reading visible. At first, it slowed down his reading rate, but as he got used to it, his reading speed eventually increased.

Use the same principle for tests where the student must read several lines or a paragraph. The window helps the youngster with TS and ADHD to focus, keep his or her place, and eliminates distraction from seeing additional material on the page.

A mother of two children with both TS and ADHD described a testing situation in which an essay on one side of a piece of paper had to be read first. Then the students were to turn the paper over and answer the questions on the back. Her youngsters lost their concentration between the reading of the essay, remembering to turn the paper over, and then answering the questions. She asked the supportive teacher to print future similar tests on two pieces of paper for her children. The teacher obliged and the youngsters performed far better without the additional distraction. This, to me, is another fine example of the benefits derived from parent and teacher working as a team.

Strengthen oral skills.

Verbal tics may interfere with a youngster's self-expression, either by interrupting his or her thought process or by drawing attention and teasing from classmates. Encourage the use of visual aids to limit verbalization in oral reports in front of the class. Be patient for the words to come, the same as you would do with a child who stuttered or had other difficulties in speaking. Insist on classroom support, courtesy, and cooperation. The students usually take their cues from their teacher. If you ignore the tics, your students also will consider them less significant.

Create writing skills support.

Writing in longhand is difficult for many children with TS because their motor tics and impaired fine motor skills make their handwriting illegible. OCD symptoms also may slow them down as they erase, rewrite, or otherwise strive for perfection while those with ADHD symptoms are plagued with impulsivity and loss of concentration as well.

In addition to problems dealing with the physical act of writing, youngsters with TS also may have difficulties with the mechanics of writing. Spelling, punctuation, and rules of grammar often are forgotten under the stress of trying to complete a writing assignment.

As writing difficulties often make note taking in class difficult, if not impossible, allow the youngster to tape lectures or select one of the more capable students in the class to use carbon paper or to permit his or her notes to be photocopied. Allotting extra time for in-class written assignments helps to reduce some of the tension that interferes with writing skills.

Have the student with TS turn in shorter written work, understanding that it may have taken that youngster more effort to produce less work. You wouldn't expect a child on crutches to join classmates for a required 50-yard dash; reconsider your requirements of "at least twenty pages" and "a minimum of one thousand words" when you are dealing with a student with TS.

Encourage the use of typewriters, computers, or tape recorders for homework. Learning to use a computer not only helps the student with TS to express his or her ideas by eliminating reliance on fine motor skills, but it also allows the student to proof his or her work through the spelling and grammar check aspects of the software program. Additional benefits derived by using word processing include giving the youngster a sense of independence along with boosting self-esteem as competency in computer use develops.

If your school system cannot provide computers for these students, find a sponsor to contribute them. Many businesses donate their older models when they purchase newer computers and/or software. Computers are not a luxury for these youngsters, but rather are an important learning tool, just as hearing aids and braille writers assist hearing and visually impaired students.

In testing situations, offer the youngster with TS a multiple-choice of "fill-in" exam, rather than one requiring essays. In multiple-choice tests, a child may have difficulty writing the word that goes in the blank. Assign numbers to each word so he or she only has to write the number for the correct answer.

The added stress from the testing environment alone may

intensify both the motor and verbal tics. Reduce the pressure by offering a quiet place in the library or an office in which to take the exam and making it an untimed test. Permit the student to take tests orally, either by giving the answer to a teacher's aide or by speaking into a tape recorder.

Boost math skills.

If the youngster crowds numbers together—which may be due to spatial problems or handwriting difficulties (or both)—have him or her use graph paper to space the numbers consistently when doing math problems. An alternative is to turn the tablet or notebook paper so the lines are vertical. That way, each number can be placed in its own column.

Allow the use of a calculator.

For homework, assign every other problem on a page rather than overwhelming the student so procrastination sets in and nothing gets done. The object of homework is to be sure a student knows the material. Often that can be achieved with fewer problems.

Reduce pressure by permitting additional time to complete work. NOTE: *Regardless of what standardized testing rules state, students with special problems (such as Tourette Syndrome) are entitled by Federal Law PL 94–142 to an adjustment of time limits.* When unrestricted time has been allowed, the teacher or monitor should write on the test paper, "Because of this student's confirmed diagnosis of a handicap, this test was completed without time limitations."

In many of the states, TS is *not* specifically listed as an "acknowledged handicap," but does come under the federal designation of "Other Health Impairments" (OHI).

BE CREATIVE WITH MOTOR ACTIVITY PROBLEMS

Permit freedom of movement.

While you can't allow a child with TS to wander at will around the classroom, you can encourage some freedom of movement. One teacher assigned a student with Tourette Syndrome and ADHD two seats in her classroom. That child was permitted to shift seats whenever he found his attention wandering or became too fidgety. Other teachers let these children squeeze erasers or rubber balls or roll bits of clay on their desks. By being permitted to express acceptable movement, many children with TS and ADHD can focus their concentration better.

Children with TS and ADHD often have a long list of "can'ts" in the classroom. They can't sit without fidgeting, can't follow through on instructions, can't finish anything, can't wait their turn, and can't play quietly. As Susan Conners put it, "To tell parents of these kids that they'd do better in class if they didn't have all these 'can'ts' is like telling the parents of a blind child, 'If your child could see he'd be a dynamite reader.' It's up to us—teachers and parents—to help that youngster learn coping skills in order to find success in school."

Allow the student to stand while working.
Standing at his desk worked successfully for Ernest Hemingway as well as for many other well-known authors. Numerous artists stand at their easel as well, so don't rule out standing for your restless student. Provide a lectern or drafting table, if possible.

Provide an escape from the classroom.
Provide opportunities for "seat breaks" by allowing the TS student to leave the classroom to get a drink of water, go to the bathroom, or run errands for you. It not only allows the youngster the freedom to give expression to the tics in relative privacy, but having the responsibility to leave when needed also boosts self-esteem by making him or her feel important.

Assign motion-oriented tasks and responsibilities.
The student with TS (and ADHD) often requires more opportunities to expend energy than the other youngsters. In the lower grades, playtime serves this purpose. In the middle and upper grades, however, other than changing classes, these children spend a great deal of time sitting. Teachers can help reduce the tension this triggers by asking that student to get up to hand out books, sharpen pencils, collect papers, etc.

In addition to providing opportunities for approved motor activity, it stimulates peer interaction, helps classmates to observe the student in a positive light, and offers the teacher a chance to praise appropriate behavior.

DEVELOP ORGANIZATIONAL PLANS

Enlist parental assistance.

Organizational breakdown occurs when one end of the "tug-of-war" lets go of the rope. You need the parents' cooperation, just as they require yours. Before implementing an organizational plan, sit down with the parents to explain what you have devised, why you came up with this particular plan, and what its objectives are. Be open to any suggestions the parents may offer. Be willing to give up pride of ownership. Never lose sight that the struggle has a purpose: to help the child with TS have the opportunity to excel in school. When dealing with parents, remember these points:

1. It's difficult for parents to have a meaningful conversation about an emotionally charged subject—their child—when sitting on Lilliputian chairs. Schedule your meeting in a conference room, a corner of the library (if it's quiet), or bring in "big people chairs" so you can speak face-to-face.

2. Although *you* are the professional when it comes to education, the parents probably are more knowledgeable about Tourette Syndrome and how it affects their child. Even if you're trained in special education, real-life situations often don't fit into textbook solutions. Each child is unique and so is the family and other circumstances. "One size fits all" doesn't work when you're dealing with how to handle TS or any other chronic disorder.

    Keep an open mind and try to learn all you can about TS. You may have another youngster with Tourette Syndrome in your classroom one day and you'll be better able to deal with that child.

3. Avoid getting defensive. While many parents probably would love for you to devote all of your time and effort to their child, most understand that you have many young-sters in your classroom and limited opportunity to deal one-on-one with their child's particular and unique prob-lem. Hear their requests and then state honestly what you feel you can and cannot do. This keeps communication lines open and prevents disappointment and resentment when you don't do what you've promised.

4. Communicate often with the parents by phone or letter. If the parents are divorced, this is especially important so the noncustodial parent doesn't get all the school information secondhand or not at all.

5. Share your observation of new tics, behavior problems, reactions to medication dosage, and so on with the parents as you may notice them first. If new tics develop that are potentially harmful to the student or classmates (physically or emotionally), discuss preventive action such as chang-ing seating, using crayons rather than pencils, or having a time-out room with the parents. Don't wait for problems to flare up before solving them.

Provide an organizational checklist.

Even commercial pilots run through a checklist before heading down the runway. Give your student a clipboard with a simplified checklist, including items that he or she has trouble remembering as well as things that you think are important. Suggestions might include homework assignment book, permission slip to be signed by a parent, gym shoes, and so on.

Some teachers include specific textbooks on the checklist; others recommend giving the student two sets of books, one for home and one for the classroom, to minimize things to be remembered.

If the youngster often forgets to bring a pencil, ask the parents to provide a box of pencils so you can quietly give him or her one. Youngsters with TS, ADHD, and OCD have so many difficulties that it seems unnecessary to expend energy arguing or penalizing the student over a pencil. Helping these children learn is a far more important issue.

Color code for immediate identification.

Just as most people recognize that red usually means "stop" or a "warning," color coding often helps children with TS with OCD and/or ADHD. It's easy to match the blue folder with the blue science book, red folder with the red math book, and so on. This prevents students from showing up with the math folder and the science book and helps them to feel organized and in control.

Equipment cupboards, lockers, and closets also can be color coded or identified with photos of what belongs inside. Most children want to become less sloppy and more organized; kids with TS and ADHD just need a little more help in doing so. (On the other hand, a youngster with TS and OCD may quickly become overly conscientious, carefully lining up each pencil and book perfectly with its neighbor and may require a reminder to begin an assignment or get to the next class.)

Use praise—either verbally or a special private signal—when things are done properly, even if it seems to take an inordinately long time. Positive reinforcement is far more effective than criticism. These youngsters want to please and don't mean to misbehave. Accent positive behavior—waiting to be called on rather than shouting out answers, handing in assignments, having a pencil and the right folder—with compliments and rewards.

Encourage these children to engage in positive self-talk, saying, "I answered all the questions you starred on my sheet," rather than, "I'm so dumb. I couldn't do all the questions." Confidence and positive self-image require careful and constant nurturing. In the beginning, it means more effort for an already busy teacher, but in the long run, it creates a more disciplined and pleasing environment, one in which *all* children have a better opportunity for learning.

CHAPTER 16

Decoding Governmental Education Guidelines[1]

In the early 1970s, when I first became aware of a disorder called Tourette Syndrome, there were fewer than a hundred cases described in the world's medical literature. We were a lonely crowd, thinking our family was the only one with this unusual problem. Because there was, as yet, no national organization to direct us to one another or to professional help, we all wandered in circles, trying first this professional, then that one, looking for answers. Each fall we prayed that our child would be assigned to an understanding and sensitive teacher with whom we could work.

Haldol was the drug of choice, but few physicians knew how to titrate it for this particular disorder. Side effects often were so severe that it almost seemed easier to suffer the symptoms than to cope with the effects of the drug controlling them.

Tourette Syndrome then was considered to be a "rare" disorder, the cause of which, according to most of the physicians, psychologists, and social workers of that era, was obviously based on "poor parenting skills." Parents were either "too permissive" or "too strict," depending on which professional you were seeing at the time.

---

[1] Much of the information used in this chapter was taken and/or adapted from materials provided by the Tourette Syndrome Association, Inc., and is used with their permission.

Not only did the parents of kids become pariahs (''Why don't you control your child?'' was the unasked as well as sometimes voiced question wherever we went), but our children often became social outcasts as well. Teachers complained that they disrupted classroom discipline (which they did), that they didn't keep up academically (which they didn't), and that they often seemed drugged and ''out of it'' (which they were). Frustrated with a system that offered no support, many parents hauled their kids out of public school, into private schools where smaller classes could give more individual attention. These educational facilities could offer that, of course, but teachers and the administration in private schools were no more knowledgeable in how to handle children with Tourette Syndrome than those in the public schools had been.

In despair, some parents opted for home schooling, recognizing that by doing so, they were reducing their youngster's opportunities for developing important social skills that would be necessary in the coming years in the real world.

In 1975, the isolation and sense that ''nobody cares'' felt by parents and families of children with TS came to an end with the passing of the Individuals with Disabilities Education Act (IDEA) by the U.S. Congress. This act, also called Public Law 94–142, the Education for All Handicapped Children Act (EAHCA), states that all children with disabilities have the right to receive ''a free, appropriate public education.''

Therefore, children with Tourette Syndrome, which *is* a handicapping condition under federal law, are guaranteed in all fifty states a ''free, appropriate public education'' in the ''least restrictive environment.'' Partial funding for necessary programs is provided by the federal government through contributions to the state. In most states, however, additional funding comes from local districts, which is why special education services may vary greatly from state to state and from district to district.

While this federal act provides for only minimum requirements for these programs, it does guarantee parents the right to work with the school in shaping approaches that will be most beneficial for their children's special needs. In addition, PL 94–142 requires that parents' consent must be received in order for the school to place their child in any program.

How to Gain Entry to "Special Education and Related Services"

When you read most materials concerning how to access the "special education and related services," it sounds more complex than it really is. Stripped of all the bureaucratic verbosity, the access ladder is as follows:

Step 1: You must notify, in writing, the school's principal or headmaster, that your child has been diagnosed with Tourette Syndrome. (You may have to digress long enough here to explain what TS is. That's where the supportive materials from the Tourette Syndrome Association come in very handy.)

Step 2: As soon as they have been notified, the school must set the evaluation process in place within a given period of time such as thirty school days. This process is conducted through a team approach, usually consisting of a psychologist, social worker, learning disabilities teacher, classroom teacher, nurse, and the case coordinator, often one of the above or a school administrator.

Your child will be given a series of standardized tests designed to pinpont specific learning difficulties, attention deficit disorder, and/or emotional problems.

While no test has been devised to state *absolutely* that a child has ADHD or TS, the diagnostic criteria mentioned in Chapter 7 are used. The tests administered by the school evaluation team—possibly including the Conners Teacher Rating Scale (CTRS), which uses direct observation by the teachers and other tests in which the child gives answers to written or visual material or responds to verbal instructions and questions—highlight the various learning problem areas such as difficulty in following directions and organizing material, faulty visual or auditory perception, impulsivity, hyperactivity, and hyperdistractibility.

Remember that positive findings for any of these learning problems do not mean that your youngster isn't smart. On the contrary, many children with Tourette Syndrome with ADHD and OCD have above average intelligence and are extremely creative. They just require a different way to process information. It's like having a computer that doesn't "read" specific commercial software programs, so the software has to be slightly customized.

In addition to the various testing procedures, you and your

spouse will be interviewed to learn more about how your child reacts in a home environment. Often behavior varies widely between home and school environments. Most children give full expression to their tics at home, while suppressing them (and suffering more stress because of the effort it requires) in school. Your child's doctors may be asked for their input too, along with a list of the medications your youngster presently is taking and their possible side effects.

This is no time to hide or dilute the truth; the purpose of this exercise is to discover what type of help your child needs in order to reach his or her potential. By lying or holding back possibly important information, you may be blocking the success of this process.

You are entitled by law to see all records pertaining to your child. Read this material over carefully and immediately point out any errors or omissions. You are allowed to delete information or purge reports when your child leaves to go to a new school.

Step 3: Within thirty days after the testing is completed, you will be notified in writing to meet with the school officials, testing team, and others concerned with your child's well-being. The time and place of the meeting must, by law, be agreeable to you. You also must be notified, in writing, of those who will be in attendance.

Although your presence is not mandatory, most parents want to be part of the process. You may request permission to tape record the meeting so that no misunderstanding occurs. (Most schools allow this.) This is especially important if only one parent attends the meeting. You also may bring someone from your local Tourette Syndrome Association or any other advocate if you so choose. If for any reason you cannot attend this or other such meetings, the Local Education Agency must arrange for a conference telephone call.

The test team will go over the test results at this meeting. Some of their language may slip into educational dialect; if you don't understand, say so. Paraphrase what you've heard to be certain you've grasped the correct meaning.

This is no time to feel defensive or feel that you have to make excuses for your child's learning and behavioral problems. Leave your ego at home. No one is blaming you for your youngster's problems. Everyone is gathered with you to help him or her succeed.

After explaining the results of the tests, the group will begin to discuss what type of assistance your child needs in order to develop to full potential. Your input is needed here too. Don't feel overwhelmed by the professional credentials of other members; you've got important credentials too. It's your child and you know him or her better than anyone, regardless of the imposing list of initials following everyone else's name.

What you and the team are working on is the design of an *individual education plan,* known by the letters IEP. This plan is carefully constructed and individualized to help your youngster fulfill both short-term and long-term goals. If there are many problems, they can't all be worked on at once. A child who gets frustrated and starts fighting with classmates must learn acceptable ways to handle his temper, for example, before he can deal with the long-term goal, which is strengthening a reading or math weakness. At times, both you and the teacher will be asked to prioritize specific areas to work on first. Take your part in formulating the IEP seriously. It's the blueprint by which your child's education foundation will be built.

Step 4: Before the IEP can be put into effect, you, as parents, must agree (or disagree) with the recommendations. If you agree (and hopefully you and the school authorities have worked together smoothly and worked out any compromises by this point), you will be asked to sign the IEP. Then, the following takes place:

1. Your child is immediately placed in the proper program, either full time or for a few hours in the school day, whatever was determined in the IEP. NOTE: Waiting lists are illegal.

If the school team indicates that your child's education needs cannot be met within the school district, the district is required to find alternative public or private placements, and to fund these services.

2. Each year you will meet with the school authorities to discuss your child's progress and to determine if changes need to

be made in the IEP for the following year. If the school doesn't notify you, you should call them.

Remember that this individual education plan is not set in stone. Give it time to work, but don't feel that you *have* to wait for the year to be up before making changes. If you ever feel that any part of the plan is ineffective, contact the school and request specific changes. Don't, however, base your decision on your child's complaint that he or she isn't learning anything, doesn't like the teacher, hates the work, and so on. Many children with TS and its concurrent disorders have difficulty in handling change. They may be rebelling at having to learn a new way of doing things, a retraining that, although painful at times, may help them greatly in the future.

If you disagree with the IEP recommendations, you can refuse to sign the document. You may bring in an education expert to make an independent evaluation and request an impartial hearing. Even if the hearing officer's decision sides with the school administration, you still have additional recourse. As these procedures may vary by state and/or be revised between the writing and the publication of this book, please contact the Tourette Syndrome Association for specific up-to-date information. (NOTE: Ask for their booklet, "Know Your Rights: Facts You Should Know About Your Rights to a Free Appropriate Public Education.")

Part V

ADULT ISSUES

CHAPTER 17

Encouraging Dating and Social Interaction

The majority of people enter their adult lives armed with social skills acquired and honed during their childhood and adolescence. The camaraderie created through participation in team sports, school plays, organizations such as scouting and religious youth groups, and peer parties taught important lessons—some painful, some painless—on what was and was not socially acceptable. Experiences gained from both shared and unrequited "puppy love" also helped to pave the way for future adult romantic relationships.

Unfortunately, for many with Tourette Syndrome, those valuable early learning years were marred by trauma created by TS symptoms at their worst. It is not uncommon for children with TS or with TS in addition to behaviors other than tics to suffer endless taunts from peers in school and on the playground; humiliation from adults, including teachers and other school personnel; and isolation from contemporaries with a resulting low self-image. While other children are finding success and self-confidence through sports and other adolescent activities, many youngsters with TS, suffering from both learning and coordination problems, are picked last for teams, embarrassed in the classroom, and struggle with behavioral difficulties generated from their ADHD and/or OCD, including flaring and uncontrollable tantrums, dangerous impulsivity, and constant feuds resulting from oppositional behavior. In addition to all these burdens, they also must cope with the ultimate curse of childhood, that of being different.

Fond memories of childhood? Never. Even if the tics have become minimal by adulthood, the scars from these painful youthful years remain. Many enter their adult years hesitant to make new acquaintances for fear of further embarrassment and defeat. Trained to be on the defensive from youth, half expecting rejection from the start, at first meeting they often appear cold, judgmental, belligerent, and withdrawn, although their newly discovered associates may not even notice what remains of the tics, or if they do, they don't mention them.

Others with TS, especially those who also have ADHD, still interact in social situations by playing the fool. Having met with their only taste of success during their school days by being the class clown, they continue to poke fun at themselves, playing practical jokes, and constantly performing, a whirlwind of madcap humor. Although some become so good at this type of sublimation that they actually become accomplished professional comedians, the majority soon wear down their peers and wear out their welcome.

Some studies suggest that many people with TS have difficulty in making and retaining close friendships with others, possibly because of a lack of experience in interacting with peers and developing social skills during childhood.

"I couldn't even hold hands with a girl when I did get a date," recalled one man with mild tics now, but who had not been diagnosed with TS until he was thirty-four. "If I did work up enough courage to take a girl's hand, my fingers wiggled constantly. They thought I was joking around and didn't like it. So . . . I stopped holding hands."

Those whose TS tics are combined with obsessive-compulsive symptomatology eventually come to realize that their unusual behavior may put unbearable strains on budding social relationships. "I know this girl really liked me," a young man admitted. "I blinked and sniffed a lot, but she seemed to understand that I couldn't help it because of my Tourette Syndrome. It was the other that must have turned her off." The "other" was his obsessive behavior, dialing her number just to hear her voice and bombarding her with gifts. Fearing rejection, he felt compelled to ensure that she was still there for him. His behavior actually forced the thing he feared most, the demise of that relationship.

Often it *is* the behavioral problem, not the verbal or motor tics, that destroys a relationships. "I didn't mind his wiping the silverware and glassware or even counting chairs whenever we went out to dinner," complained a young woman who had gone out with a teacher who had both TS and OCD, "but he kept touching people on their shoulder or arm, then asking them if he could 'even it up' by touching them on the other side. I felt as though I was in a television sit-com."

Other men and women had ended relationships with people with TS because of the violent outbursts of temper or the impulsivity, which sometimes can be downright dangerous. Because many young men and women with TS, ADD, and OCD are "dating impaired," that is, they have little experience in dealing socially with the opposite sex, they not only suffer from extremely low self-confidence levels but they also have poor social judgment. Like a child prattling on and exposing the family's dirty linen, these individuals may reveal too much about themselves on the first date or ask questions of their companion that are far too intimate for this initial situation.

Sometimes those with TS are able to see the humor in these situations themselves and can help defuse most awkward moments. Others, however, who demand perfection from themselves as well as others, may see no humorous side. While encouragement and training may be able to help this young adults to "lighten up" a little, we all innately possess (or do not possess) our own unique sense of humor. It is difficult to try to train someone to react in a way that is not in his or her nature.

For those entering the adult years devoid of much practical experience in dealing with social interaction, the local or regional Tourette Syndrome Support Group offers a safe and supportive peer group. (Contact the national TSA office to learn the location of one in your area.) Here, among those with familiar symptoms and stories, a wavering self-image can be nurtured.

According to Carolyn R. Shaffer and Kristin Anundsen, coauthors of *Creating Community Anywhere: Finding Support and Connection in a Fragmented World,* "support groups allow you to be yourself, to tell the truth about both your weaknesses and your strengths. . . . You also learn how to listen to others without judging them and offer help without trying to fix them.''

Emily Kelman-Bravo, a clinical social worker and director of TSA's New York City Counseling Program, runs numerous peer groups for youngsters and adults with TS. "I believe the support offered by these groups is extremely helpful," she said, "but I think it's also important to be challenged by someone with the same problem. For example, if someone in the group complains that his boss is always down on him, constantly criticizing, a peer can say, 'Hey, don't you think it's odd that you've said that about *every* boss you've had on every job? Could all your bosses really be wrong? Maybe the problem is with *you*.'

"It's empowering to learn from others," Kelman-Bravo added. "Many of the adults in the groups I've run have had *no* contact with others who have TS. They've been terribly isolated. Often they find out things about themselves that they never knew were Tourette related . . . like having overwhelming rages or unbearable depression.''

"I felt so relieved when someone else said they felt these rages," a young man confided. "I never told anyone how this deep anger raged inside me, how I had to run away to hide so I could hit the wall until my fists bled. When another guy in my group described this exact experience, I cried. I felt as though someone, at last, had built a bridge to my island and I was no longer alone.''

"These sessions often are extremely therapeutic," Kelman-Bravo said. "Newcomers who have just been diagnosed—and remember, they've had TS since they were kids and are now, in their adult years, just learning that what's wrong with them has a name—sometimes come in a little uptight. Then they hear the others joking, actually laughing at their own tics and everyone else's tics. It isn't gallows humor. Some of the tics are very funny. We had one man who repeated lines from commercials. It's very therapeutic to be able to see that humor. It's very healing.''

An additional benefit from meeting with others with TS is that people share methods they have used successfully to control behavior problems. While there is a great variability with TS, some suggestions appear to be almost universally helpful, such as controlling temper outbursts by using a punching bag, counting to ten before blowing up, walking around the block to cool off, and even learning how to apologize to one's boss, coworkers, peers, friends, and relatives if none of these modalities prove effective in staving off a tantrum.

Those who can't handle the frustration of standing in line without losing their temper learn avoidance techniques, such as going at a quieter time of day or midweek rather than on Friday.

"Adults need to feel they have some control," Kelman-Bravo stated. "They learn many positive procedures from those who have 'been there' in their group meetings."

While researchers have documented the effectiveness of peer support groups, it's important for members of such groups to guard against meetings becoming merely gripe sessions.

CHAPTER 18

Developing and Maintaining a Satisfying Intimate Relationship

As a nation we seem to be preoccupied with matters of sex, flocking to movies showing graphic scenes of sexual activity, supporting cable stations presenting what used to be called pornographic material, and purchasing millions of dollars worth of books and magazines crammed with photos and descriptions of writhing bodies locked in carnal combat. Nevertheless, we are peculiarly puritanical when it comes to discussing our personal sexual lives, even with our doctor.

Some of that reluctance may come from our sensing that our physician is uncomfortable in talking about sex. Many adults with Tourette Syndrome admitted that they also felt discomfort when trying to talk about sexual matters with their physician.

"It embarrasses me to talk about my sex life," a forty-year-old businessman admitted. "My wife's understanding, but I jerk, hoot, and yelp while we're making love. Unfortunately, it's not from the throes of passion. I'm afraid it isn't too romantic. I don't know if the doctor could help. Most of the ones I've even hinted about the problem to quickly changed the subject. I've never felt comfortable pursuing the matter with any of them."

A younger man with TS and OCD confided that, while he was pleased with the way Prozac helped him to control symptoms of his OCD, he was disturbed about one of the side effects his doctor had failed to even mention: he had lost all interest in having sex. "Because of my tics and compulsions, I never had any girlfriends in high school," he murmured sadly. "Now that my symptoms are somewhat under control, I do date a little, but because of the medication, I've no interest in making love. I sometimes wonder if the trade-off is worth it.''

When I asked if he had discussed his lack of sex drive with his doctor, he shook his head. ''No, I can't talk to him about things like that. He didn't even think it was important enough to tell me that Prozac can cause that. I'd feel odd talking to him about my lack of a sex life.''

The best course of action for this young man is to see his doctor immediately and begin discussions with him. If he isn't comfortable with his physician, he should seek out a trained social worker, psychologist, or a member of the clergy in whom he can confide. The situation need not be hopeless or permanent. There are several specific antidotes, such as yohimbine or periactin, to counter this effect of Prozac (which is shared by Zoloft and Paxil). Also, medications *can* be titrated to reduce, though not necessarily eradicate, potentially disturbing side effects. In addition, there may be other chemical combinations that could be as effective or almost as effective without similar side effects.

Each person is different and reacts differently to medication. But sexual problems should never be accepted without question or considered unimportant. Sex is an important part of one's life. If you had problems with any other aspect of daily life you'd discuss it with someone who could help you. Do the same with your sexual life.

If your doctor doesn't feel at ease discussing sexual issues and cannot refer you to a therapist or other specialist who may be able to help, contact the American Association of Sex Educators, Counselors, and Therapists (AASECT). This is an association of certified professionals, trained in the field of sex education and sex counseling.

For a list of names of qualified sex therapists in your state or province, send a stamped, self-addressed #10 envelope (the long narrow kind) along with a check for $3 made out to AASECT. Mail it to:

AASECT
Suite 1717
435 N. Michigan Avenue
Chicago, IL 60611

Do *not* send a letter describing your particular problems as this is only a referral agency. If you want lists for more than one state or province, send an additional $3 per list and write the name of the state or province on the lower left corner of your return envelope.

All Intimacy Is Not Sex

Although sexual intimacy may be a part of a relationship, it is not the only part, nor is it, say many men and women, the most important part.

To be satisfying, an intimate relationship requires honesty, trust, and consideration. It also demands time to grow and develop. Unfortunately, time is often a most scarce commodity when a couple is dealing with one or more children with Tourette Syndrome, especially if OCD and/or ADHD is involved. By the time the parents have worked all day, come home to fix dinner, then struggle through refereeing fights between siblings, homework hassles, and putting hyperactive kids to bed, they themselves collapse into bed.

Sexual intimacy also can be threatened when one of the partners has TS and suffers from a decreased sex drive or ability because of medication side effects, fear of pregnancy and the possibility of having a child with TS, or a general sense of being unlovable. Both foreplay and sexual intercourse may be abandoned—either due to fear of failure and/or rejection or disinterest.

Intimacy does not need to be—and should not be—neglected. There are many ways to affirm your love and feelings for one another without actually having sexual intercourse. That's where honesty and trust come in. There needs to be open communication, so that either spouse feels comfortable and nonthreatened by saying, "We don't have to make love, but I need some holding time," or "please just hold me." The value isn't minimized just because you had to ask for it. A caring hug can soothe both the "hugger" and the "huggee," reaffirming the relationship. It's a positive stroke for both.

There are other strokes that say, "I love you," other than having intercourse. Massaging one another, holding hands, and old-fashioned "necking" give the gift of touch to both participants. So does sitting side by side, walking together, or sharing a sunset.

Remember when you're giving out hugs to share some with your kids, especially the one with TS with OCD and/or ADHD. It's easy for these youngsters to feel unloved and unwanted. Their self-esteem is battered at school, they often seem to be in trouble with their siblings, and everyone keeps pointing out all the things they're doing wrong. Their behavioral problems make people—even their parents, at times—draw away. A sincere hug and a kiss can let them know that they're cared for too.

CHAPTER 19

Determining and Finding the "Right" Job

As soon as the shock of the diagnosis of Tourette Syndrome sinks in, the next thought many parents have is, "What will become of my child? Will he (or she) ever be able to hold down a job?"

The answer, of course, is a resounding "yes." Many people with TS have mild or no obvious symptoms once they reach adulthood. Their employers and coworkers may never realize that these individuals have anything wrong with them at all. Even those with moderate and more severe tics can and do hold down permanent jobs as well as enjoy extremely rewarding careers.

There are adults with Tourette Syndrome teaching in our schools, treating and operating on patients, and playing professional sports. There are actors, bankers, and clerks; lawyers, musicians, nurses, and officers in the military; researchers, social workers, and therapists. You can run through the entire alphabet of employment opportunities and probably find someone with Tourette Syndrome working in each category.

Ironically, some of the "problems" identified with TS during childhood, when a youngster is confined by a restrictive school setting, may be transformed into assets for adults in selective career fields. Musicians, actors, and salespeople have often harnessed the excess energies created by TS along with OCD and/or ADHD with much success in bolstering their performances; authors and artists have used their distractibility and "different" way of looking at a subject to achieve great acclaim in their creative endeavors. Swiss psychiatrist and psychologist Carl Jung praised this type of inattention, daydreaming, and risk-taking behavior by saying, "Without this playing with fantasy, no creative work has ever yet come to birth."

Inventor Thomas Alva Edison, who only had three months of formal education and found that to be "distracting," proved that his inability to concentrate on one subject for any length of time actually led him into greater experimentation and success. At his death in 1931, 1,093 patents were registered in his name, among them the electric light bulb, the first automatic telegraph, and the phonograph. Not bad for a kid who couldn't sit still.

People with OC traits along with their TS often discover that they can utilize their perfectionistic tendencies by channeling them into successful organizational skills, creating greater advantage in the business arena and helping them to achieve much success. Super organizers turn their talents into an entrepreneurial enterprise helping others to become more efficient.

Although it seems as though some types of work may not be particularly well suited for those with severe tics, ADHD, and/or OCD, for any specific occupation I might mention there are bound to be a few people who are the exception and could prove that they are overwhelmingly successful in that particular field of endeavor. Those choices must be made on an individual basis, not by assuming (or by accepting someone else's assumption) that you can't do a particular task because of your TS.

Unfortunately, those whose tics follow them into adulthood (possibly accompanied by ADHD and/or OCD) often bring the same difficulties to their job that made the school years difficult for them. They still may find it hard to pay attention and follow instructions. Those in positions of responsibility may become distracted, give incomplete instructions to their staff, or forget what directives they issued the day before. They lose original papers, forget major appointments, and miss important deadlines. As with their school years, their low frustration level may cause them to frequently lose their tempers and tell off the boss or coworkers, or to just give up and quit. Some of these individuals hop from job to job, vainly searching for that illusive perfect job.

Yet many of the same supportive techniques that helped these people cope with school could also be effective in the work force. Often, however, these procedures are forgotten or ignored. Mommy is no longer there to intercede. Unless the parents have helped their child develop independence and a strong sense of self-confidence, the young adult may not be organized or responsible enough to follow through or even to remember what worked in high school or college.

What Is the "Right" Job?

Numerous adults with Tourette Syndrome who have developed their own successful businesses and careers suggest steering young people with TS into jobs with flexibility. "Having to adhere to a strict time schedule may create too much stress," a public relations consultant advised. "Tension triggers tic intensity. Then too, sometimes my compulsions to check all the locks on the doors and windows before leaving home make me late getting to the office. If I knew I had to punch a time clock, I'd go berserk."

Yet, having said that, many employees with TS do work successfully within a time-intensive system, reporting that the structure and guidelines actually helped to keep them focused. Whereas one adult with TS and OCD advised, "Stay away from jobs where you have to follow specific orders exactly. The military, for instance, would be an awful choice," another adult who also had TS and OCD reported that his life in the military was ideal for him. "My OCD makes me the perfect officer," he said. "I do everything by the book."

Certainly this divergence of viewpoints suggests that "Know yourself" is of utmost importance before starting a job search. Each person with TS is an individual and the variations in tics and their severity fluctuate wildly as they also wax and wane. What another person considers to be an ideal job may not work for you and your particular needs.

If you have an attention deficit disorder as well, you may find difficulty concentrating or focusing on particular aspects of a job. "I can't follow instructions," a thirty-year-old man said simply.

"I try, but it's like it was in school. Hopeless. I'm as frustrated now as I was then." His present job—which he enjoys—is working for a landscaper, where his immediate superior gives him one task at a time. When he completes that, she gives him the next one. "She's really patient and understanding," he said. "Her brother had ADHD too."

Select jobs that play to your strengths, not your weaknesses. If time pressure makes your symptoms worse, don't interview for a job on a newspaper or ad agency, where everything needs to be done yesterday and deadlines are a fact of life. Similarly, working on an assembly line may be extremely frustrating and even hazardous for someone with impulsivity who also is highly distractible.

"I found that being my own boss worked best for me," a thirty-something artist announced. "Although I'm an expert at holding back my tics, I'm very self-conscious about people noticing them. I always have to be in control. I have to have structure to cope. Working for myself put me in charge and I like that."

Others agree with her. "Try to get a job situation in which you call the shots," a physician with TS advised. "If you have confrontational behavior, it puts you at risk. If you're easily ticked off by authority figures, structure your life to avoid them as much as possible."

A truck driver with coprolalia found his job was perfect for him as he worked alone much of the time and could suppress his tics when he had to interact with others. Another called his work as a fishing guide "ideal," saying. "Nobody minds my tics as long as they're catching fish."

There's no doubt that finding a job that fits your particular needs as well as it being one that you also enjoy helps to reduce the stress level in your life. This is important for everyone, but even more so for the person with Tourette Syndrome. Whether it's stuffing envelopes and answering phone calls, selling a product or arguing a legal case in court, the hours you spend at work, the coworkers with whom you interact, and the environment that surrounds you all affect your personal well-being. Consider your potential job carefully.

Where to Begin

Once you have carefully assessed your interests, needs, and abilities, you're ready to zero in on finding a job. Be flexible. According to the *Dictionary of Occupational Titles*, there are more than twenty thousand different types of jobs.

How do you learn about potential job openings? There are a number of ways. Volunteer work is a good way to get your foot into the job market.

Many people achieve permanent employment from a temporary job. In fact, according to the National Association of Temporary Services (NATS), approximately half of all temporary workers gain permanent positions in the firms in which they worked. Temporary jobs also are a good option for those who have ADD because they can move on to a new job with new coworkers if they become restless. Many businesses prefer hiring "temps" because they can expand their staff for busy seasons and easily reduce them when things get slow. Best of all, many temp services train their clients on computers and other business machines.

You also could begin your job search by checking the want ads in the classified section of the newspaper, although that's usually not the best way, as 75–80 percent of jobs are filled *before* they're listed in the newspaper. Be cautious of ads offering fantastically high salaries for what seems like minimal qualifications. They probably *are* too good to be true.

One of the best avenues to travel in your job hunt is networking, talking to everyone you know and describing the type of job you desire. Some individuals, especially those who had a difficult time with peer relationships in their adolescence and high year school years, may feel uncomfortable about networking, seeing it as asking favors. They may lack self-confidence. "What if I ask if they can help me and they say 'no'?" one young woman asked. The answer to that, of course, is that (1) if they say "no," they say "no" and you're no worse off than you were before, and (2) they *may* say "yes." If they do, prepare for the interview, recognizing that it may be the one that gets you a job.

Connections usually won't *get* you a job, but they may open a few doors to help you get an interview. Even if you don't get *that* job, the interviewer may know who else is looking for somebody with your qualifications. Let as many people as possible know you're looking for a job. Something may click.

One of my children got her first teaching position because a coworker at her temporary job with a building company said his mother, an elementary school principal, was interviewing teachers that week. He hounded her until she made the phone call, which led to the interview, and ultimately, the job offer. She's now a tenured teacher at the same school.

There also are private employment agencies that screen applicants for some employers. Check references carefully before you get involved as all agencies may not have the same standards. Ask who is paying the fee for a particular job. In some cases, it is the employer; in others, it is the applicant. If you don't want a percentage of your paycheck taken out each month for the employment agency's fee, ask for information on fee-paid positions only.

Public employment agencies do not charge for their services and have information concerning government jobs. Check your phone book for their location.

In addition, vocational rehabilitation services are available in every state to all adults with handicapping conditions including Tourette Syndrome. (These services are known by various names such as VR, OVR, or VESID. Check your phone book for the district office nearest you.) The services include testing to determine your occupational strengths and weaknesses, counseling, vocational training, books and necessary equipment, and job referrals. Make your requests as specific as possible so the counselor can be of greatest benefit to you.

Check your library or bookstore for titles of books specifically written to help you analyze your abilities and interests and find the right job.

Perhaps one of the best books in this field is *What Color Is Your Parachute?* by Richard Nelson Bolles, originally published in 1970, but revised annually. The 1990 and 1991 editions included a special section titled "Job-Hunting Tips for the So-called Handicapped." More recent editions have excluded it.

Another book offering meaningful suggestions to those with TS who are job hunting is *Successful Job Search Strategies for the Disabled* by Jeffrey G. Allen, J.D., C.P.C.

What Is an Office?

Never assume that you can't get a job because your symptoms make it difficult for you to work alongside coworkers or in an office environment. Today there are many variations in what constitutes a business office. It could be your car, home, or even your boat as modern telecommunications allow employees the opportunity to perform their jobs from nontraditonal locations thanks to computers, fax machines, modems, and other electronic devices unheard of just a few decades ago. Look for any of the "working-at-home" or "your-home-office"-type books at your library or bookstore. Three helpful books are *Working from Home* by Paul and Sarah Edwards, *The Home Office* by Peg Contrucci, and *Working at Home: Is It for You?* by William Atkinson. As this is a growing market, similar books are released on the subject continually.

In addition to new *places* to work, there are modern, less rigid *methods* of doing one's job. Two of these innovative techniques that might prove helpful are job sharing and flextime. In job sharing, two people divide up one job. Teachers and salespeople often manage this successfully, with one teacher or salesperson handling the job in the morning and the other taking charge in the afternoon. It also could be a shared job with one worker covering Monday, Tuesday, and half of Wednesday, and the partner assuming responsibility for the remainder of the week.

Although the salary and benefits are also halved, this nontraditional type of employment might be a good option for someone testing the waters, or someone who has trouble staying on task for five days at a time. Many employers are already familiar with job sharing, but you may have to convince others that it can work. Communication is vital to the success of job sharing, however, so don't try it if you have difficulty being organized enough to tell your partner what you've done and what is yet to be handled.

Flextime also has proven to be successful for many office workers who prefer to select those forty hours a week that best suit them and their schedule. It might appeal to those whose vocal tics disturb coworkers during regular hours as they could report to work just as the others are leaving for the day.

In addition, there are a host of jobs for those who prefer the out-of-doors or other environments, or those who prefer nontraditional work. Be creative. Whatever your disability from TS, ADHD, or OCD, there *are* job opportunities and possibilities for you.

Why You Need to Work

Why is getting and holding a job so important? Because work is what adults do. Just as school is the child's work, so work is the job of the adult. It not only gives structure to our day—especially important to those who have ADD as well—but it also affects many aspects of our lives. Our work offers us the opportunity for socializing and getting to know a variety of people. The right job helps to build confidence in our abilities and to develop self-esteem. It creates a sense of pride in having produced something worthwhile. And every bit as important as the other benefits, employment also offers financial independence.

But when an adult is unable to get or hold a job, which sometimes happens to those with Tourette Syndrome, the world shrinks dramatically. First of all, the usual adult role must be redefined. Most of us get a sense of identity through our work. We are writers, teachers, taxi cab drivers, real estate salespeople, accountants, or chefs. If we don't work or we have difficulty holding a job, it may have damaging effects on our self-image because, rightly or wrongly, we don't have that job label with which to describe ourselves.

By necessity, adult children who don't work will probably remain financially dependent on their parents. Maturity is delayed or indefinitely postponed. This creates an endless circle of dependency, as well as possible resentment by the parents, who thought their child-rearing responsibilities were about to end; by the adult child, who wants the normal independence that comes with his or her age; and even by younger siblings who may still be at home, and who expected their time in the spotlight, at last.

Financial dependency also fosters a lack of confidence in one's ability. What's more, lack of financial independence combined with a probable history in adolescence of poor social skills may delay the realization of other adult roles, such as dating, courtship, marriage, and possibly parenthood.

Probably the most serious outcome of not working, however, is that in our culture adults are *supposed* to work. Only those who are old, ill, and infirm are easily excused from work responsibilities. When an adult with Tourette Syndrome doesn't work, the implication to others is that he or she really is "different" (i.e., sick). It also reinforces the negative "poor me" connotations in the mind (and actions) of the person with TS.

Can Parents Help?

Parents with adult children who may be reluctant to test the job market must be firm, encouraging, and supportive. They should be unified in their desire to help their grown offspring locate some type of employment. A volunteer position or a part-time job, even one with no room for growth is desirable over the alternatives, that of becoming a recluse and moping in one's room, "vegging out" in front of the television, or hanging out with other unemployed adults. Even an entry-level job allows the person to test the waters and gain some semblance of confidence. Getting dressed and going to work bolsters self-respect, which reinforces itself.

Never ridicule any job opportunity or fret that it is beneath your adult child's ability. It may, of course, be just that, but it also may be the stepping stone toward freedom and a sense of confidence that will lead to his or her applying for a more rigorous employment challenge the next time.

CHAPTER 20

Knowing Your Employment Rights[1]

Before sending in your resume or calling to set up an interview for a job, you must know your legal rights concerning employment. Prospective employers may not be aware of these rights, which are guaranteed to you by federal law, and you may have to (gently) educate them.

As part of the Rehabilitation Act of 1973, Congress passed Section 504, the first federal civil rights law protecting the rights of individuals with handicaps. It provided that "no otherwise qualified individual with handicaps in the United States . . . shall, solely by reason of . . . handicap, be excluded from the participation in, be denied the benefits of, or be subjected to discrimination under any program or activity receiving Federal financial assistance."

It also states, "No qualified handicapped person shall, on the basis of handicap, be subjected to discrimination in employment under any program or activity that receives or benefits from Federal financial assistance. Recipients (of the Federal financial assistance) may not limit, segregate or classify applicants or employees in any way that adversely affects their opportunities or status because of handicaps."

Agencies not abiding by this regulation are in danger of losing their federal funding. Although these programs primarily included schools, libraries, and other state agencies receiving

---

[1] Much of the information used in this section was taken and/or adapted from material supplied by the U.S. Equal Employment Opportunity Commission.

monies from the federal government, it enables children and adults with TS to receive accommodations in order to continue their education.

The Americans with Disabilities Act of 1990 (ADA) was enacted to eliminate discrimination in all areas, not just those that were federally funded. This act makes it unlawful to discriminate in employment against a qualified individual with a disability.

Note the inclusion of the word *qualified*. Legally, it means that if your ability, education, and training are superior to that of other applicants, they cannot be hired instead of you merely because you have TS and your tics may bother others. However, in practice, what constitutes being qualified is often in the eyes of the beholder. That subjective judgment is sometimes used to prevent the hiring of a person with Tourette Syndrome or any other noticeable disability. If you could prove this, of course, it would be illegal, and could be reported to the U.S. Equal Employment Opportunity Commission (EEOC) and your state and local civil rights enforcement agencies that work with the EEOC. Unfortunately, there's often a gray area as to what makes one person qualifiable, or more qualifiable, than another.

Nevertheless, the law is on your side. Plain and simple, the section of the ADA that deals with job discrimination makes it illegal for all employers (including state and local government agencies) with fifteen or more employees to practice job discrimination against people with disabilities.

According to the Americans with Disabilities Act, "An employer is required to provide a reasonable accommodation to a qualified applicant or employee with a disability *unless* [my italics] the employer can show that the accommodation would be an undue hardship—that is, would require significant difficulty or expense."

That means that your employer would have to accommodate your symptoms by moving your desk so your arm tic wouldn't cause you to clobber your coworker; rearrange your work table so it would face inward, rather than toward a window, another employee, or other distracting view; or allow you to use a typewriter or computer (providing one was available), if your motor tics caused your handwriting to be illegible. Your employer would not, however, have to build a special soundproof office for you (but would have to give it to you if one were available) if your vocal tics made it difficult for other employees to perform their work.

Your employer *is* required to provide whatever accommodations are required for you to perform your job *unless* the cost of doing so is an undue hardship. If that's the case, you still have the choice of providing the accommodation yourself or of paying for the portion of the accommodation that is the hardship. By law, your employer cannot lower your salary in order to make up the cost of providing a reasonable accommodation for your disability.

Never be afraid to ask for accommodations in order to fulfill the requirements of a job. Almost everyone who works makes minor accommodations without even thinking about it. I'm left-handed. In every job I've ever held, one of the first things I do after sitting down at my desk is to move the telephone to the right side of the desk so that I can pick up the receiver with my right hand and take notes with my left. Some of the changes you may require for a particular job—a headset on the telephone, moving a desk, or posting written instructions in order of priority—may be no more complicated than that.

Determine what accommodations you'll need in a particular job and their cost in order to reassure prospective employers that they can easily make these adaptations so that you can do a good job.

Additional ADA requirements make it unlawful to discriminate in all employment practices including not only recruitment and hiring, but also job assignments, payment, layoff, firing, training, promotions, benefits, leave, and all other employment-related activities. It is unlawful for an employer to retaliate against you for asserting your rights under the ADA. The act also protects you if you are a victim of discrimination because of your family, business, social, or other relationship or association with an individual with a disability.

The TSA offers materials that explain your legal rights in more detail. Use this information to support your position, if necessary, rather than getting into an adversarial situation with a prospective employer. If you want a particular job badly enough to interview for it, it's probably not a good idea to start off by antagonizing the person who can give it to you. Knowing that you are protected from discrimination by the federal government should give you a sense of confidence and the interviewers some concern if they consider you qualified for a job, but hesitate offering it because of your tics or other disabilities created by TS.

Be aware that the ADA also outlaws discrimination against individuals with disabilities in state and local government services, public accommodations, transportation, and telecommunications.

If differences should arise over the interpretation or implementation of the ADA, your first step should be to try to negotiate and find a mutually acceptable solution. If this alternative fails, however, file a written complaint with the:

Equal Employment Opportunity Commission
1801 L Street, N.W.
Washington, DC 20507
(800) 669-EEOC

If you're dissatisfied with the resolution of the matter by the EEOC, you have yet another recourse. As a private party, you also have the right to bring a lawsuit against an employer or potential employer. You should, however, enlist the services of a knowledgeable attorney who specializes in rights of the handicapped if you decide to utilize this option.

Contact your local or state Bar Association for information. Your Legal Aid Society or American Civil Liberties Union can help you if you are unable to pay for legal counsel.

Much of this material is confusing. But it's important in order to take advantage of those laws already in existence to help you and to determine what yet needs to be accomplished. Don't be surprised if many of the officials—state, local, and federal as well—don't totally comprehend how these laws pertain to you as a person with TS.

The U.S. Equal Employment Opportunity Commission has material on job rights for disabled people for both employers and employees. Write to the EEOC and ask for their free booklets.

In summary, remember that the Americans with Disabilities Act (ADA) offers you or a loved one with TS this "Bill of Rights":

- The right not to be discriminated against on the basis of being regarded as a person with a disability.
- The right to be judged on your own merits.
- The right not to be screened out of employment on the basis of a disability.
- The right to reveal to an employer a disabling condition without being discriminated against.
- The right to be tested fairly as an applicant for a job.
- The right to request and be provided with reasonable accommodations that are not an undue hardship on an employer.
- The right not to be disqualified in employment based on the inability to perform nonessential job functions.
- The right not to be limited, segregated, or classified as a person with a disability.
- The right not to be asked about a disabling condition.

CHAPTER 21

Interviewing

Should you tell that you have TS or not tell? The decision can be a difficult and somewhat frightening one. The response by fifty adults and young people in their late teens to this question was evenly split. The "You might as well tell. They'll eventually find out" group relied on the "Honesty is the best policy" theory. They admitted, however, that making this determination was aided by knowing that they also had the legal clout of the ADA behind them, which makes it illegal to refuse to hire a qualified person based on his or her disability. They also were aware that the ADA prohibits an interviewer from asking what type of treatment and/or medication you're receiving.

"I definitely think you should tell a prospective boss," a city employee with TS added. "Employers are required to provide reasonable accommodation only for the physical and mental limitations of qualified individuals with disabilities of which they are aware. If you don't tell them beforehand, how do you know that they won't claim it's an 'undue hardship'? You might as well know up front." This young man's motor tics included a frequent tugging on both of his earlobes. He required a speaker phone in order to handle in a timely manner the hundreds of calls his department received. His immediate supervisor easily agreed to this accommodation at the time of the interview.

Although you legally do not need to discuss your disability—only how you can do a particular job—many adults in the "Do tell" category suggested that the best way to inform a prospective employer about your disorder is to be matter-of-fact about it. Have an information sheet with pertinent questions and answers or one of the TSA's brochures available, and say something like, "The tics you see are symptoms of a neurological disorder I have called Tourette Syndrome. They are involuntary, but don't interfere with my ability to perform this job. I'll be happy to answer any questions you may have."

Chances are you won't get many questions. If you do, it's an opportunity to educate the interviewer. Don't overexplain or use complex medical terminology. Just give necessary information that pertains to any potential accommodations you may need and go on to discuss how well qualified you are for the job. Your employer doesn't need to know that the tics worsen in the theater, for example, unless you're being interviewed for the position of usher or actor.

Some people suggested that you wait until the second interview or when you get a job offer before explaining about TS. The majority, however, felt that if you don't talk about it up front, chances are there wouldn't be a second interview and/or job offer, especially if your tics are particularly severe.

"If you're sitting there slapping the arm of the chair and hooting, and you don't mention why you're doing it, I think it makes things worse," a lanky young woman said as she displayed those very tics. "The poor interviewer is thinking, 'My God, she must be crazy.' Why make it worse for yourself? I always tell about my TS and OCD and then show my references. I'm a good secretary. I type 75 words per minute, my shorthand speed is 110, and I know Word, WordPerfect, and Lotus 1-2-3. I'm great at details. My tics don't interfere with my work in any way, so why make them seem like stumbling blocks? Of course I tell."

The "Don't tell" faction, obviously comprised largely of people who had few obvious tics or who could mask or suppress their symptoms, argued that you should withhold the fact that you have TS until you are hired. They also were well aware of the ADA guidelines that make it illegal for an employer to ask about the nature or severity of your disability. (An employer *can*, however, ask if you can perform the duties of the job with or without reasonable accommodation and can also ask you to describe or demonstrate how, with or without accommodation, you will perform the duties of the job.)

If you decide not to tell a prospective employer about your TS during an interview and you get the job, what happens if you display symptoms at work? The next chapter offers some suggestions by people who have been there.

Preparing for the Interview

• *Learn something about the company* before *the interview.* I was amazed to hear one of my son's college friends say as he was running off to an interview late in his senior year that he had no idea what the company did. (He didn't get the job.) On the other hand, when you have some background on a prospective employer you can say, "How did you expand your button market so successfully?" or "How does the summer white sale compare to the Christmas sales in volume?" The interviewer knows you're interested enough in his or her company to do your homework. You've also touched on a subject close to the interviewer's heart: *the company.* That has to be a plus for you. Your local library, newspaper, and Chamber of Commerce can give you a wealth of information on a particular company. You also can ask the company's public relations department for brochures, press kits, or annual reports. If it's a small business, check the newspaper for ads to get an idea what they sell, how, and when.

• *Never walk into an interview cold.* To do so wastes both your time and that of the one doing the interview. Put yourself in prospective employers' shoes and ask yourself what they would want to learn about you. Interview yourself. What do you do well? What is your strong suit? Your weakest trait? What skills needed for this particular job do you still lack? How can you develop them?

In many cases, what you learn about yourself might mean revising your resume to fit a particular situation. If you're an artist, for example, and you're applying for the position of artist in residence with a private school, you'd want to highlight your teaching experience, your past work as a counselor for kids at an art camp, and the mobile canvas project that you created and brought into the inner city. If you also are interviewing for a job working with retirees in an assisted congregant living facility, you'd rewrite your resume to stress your art projects for Meals on Wheels, the art lessons you gave at a geriatric recreation center, and then your teaching experience. Keep your resume flexible, on a computer, rather than having hundreds of copies of identical ones printed.

• *Never underestimate the importance of practicing your interview techniques.* It helps you to be prepared for the real event. Use visualization to see yourself walking into the room, shaking hands with the interviewers, and selling yourself for a particular job. Run that mental tape over and over until you feel it's set. That's why the top free-throw shooters in basketball practice almost daily until shooting a free-throw becomes almost second nature. Their body is trained to react; they're focused. They visualize themselves at the free-throw line and mentally picture themselves making each basket. Public speakers and top salespeople incorporate the same mental preparation into their planning before making presentations. It may seem effortless when you hear them, but that's because they practiced.

Interviewing is no different. With practice, you don't have to worry how you look, answer questions, shake hands, or even walk out of the door. Rehearsing makes you more composed. When you're low-key about your TS, a prospective employer may not think it's such a big deal either. Ask a friend to role-play with you. Better yet, try to get someone to videotape your role-playing so you can watch yourself objectively and correct any mistakes.

• *If you have the option, schedule the interview at the best time for you.* Some people with TS who take medication are groggy in the morning from it and say their mind feels fuzzy. Others are more affected later in the day. You may be asked for a time preference for the interview, so be kind to yourself. Don't fight your body's rhythm. You'll just create more stress, which probably means more tics as well. Practice relaxation techniques or self-hypnosis before leaving for the interview. If your compulsions slow you down, making you check and recheck your briefcase, the resume, and your car keys, start extra early so you're not late.

• *Always be on time for your interview*. If you aren't sure of the location, check it out a few days before. Even if you're delayed because of something out of your control, you'll still have to start the interview with an apology. Not good. Plan to arrive at least ten minutes early so you have time to compose yourself and your thoughts.

• *Dress for business*. You're always safest to wear a coat and tie (if you're male) and a tailored suit or dress (if you're female). Wear your interview outfit for your role-playing to be sure it's comfortable. If something around your neck makes your tics more intense, get a larger-size collar and tie the tie loosely.

Don't wear jewelry other than a watch and ring. Women shouldn't wear gaudy or jangling earrings; men should refrain from earrings altogether, unless applying for a job in the creative professions where they're more accepted.

• *Watch your posture*. Walk in with a confident manner. If your interviewer offers to shake hands, do so with a firm handshake.

If asked to sit, do so without collapsing as though you are exhausted. If the chair is too deep for you, sit midway back on the seat, rather than slumping or having your legs dangle. If you're a finger-tapper, try to hold your hands in your lap, rather than letting them dance on the arms of your chair.

• *Try to make the interviewer comfortable with your symptoms*. He or she may not be an accomplished interviewer and may find your tics distracting or worrisome. You want an interviewer to concentrate on you, not your tics.

• *Be positive*. Talk about what you can and have accomplished before mentioning any accommodations you may need.

• *Don't be defensive and start quoting your legal rights (although you should know what they are)*.

• *Be honest*. Don't claim credentials that you don't have or say that you're good at details if you're not. You'll quickly be found out.

• *Keep the discussion focused on the job, not on your TS.*

• *Maintain eye contact, but don't stare.* Don't worry if you have an eye tic. If it's severe, casually mention that you have TS and that's why you're blinking. Although it's illegal for an interviewer to ask about your tics, you may sense that he or she would like to know more about TS. If you feel comfortable and want to share this information, it's a good opportunity to briefly describe what it is, stressing that having TS in no way affects your work or ability. But it's *your* decision whether or not to mention it. While the interviewer cannot initiate conversation about your tics, he or she can ask how you would handle a particular task that is important to the prospective job.

• *Ask intelligent questions.* Don't feel as though you *have* to ask questions and certainly don't ask those you should know the answer to, such as "What products does your company manufacture?" Don't give lengthy answers to questions posed to you. The interview probably will be less than 30 minutes, so use the allotted time to your benefit. If you don't know how to answer a particular question, admit it. Don't try to fake it. There's nothing wrong with saying, "I don't know how I'd handle that. I'd have to know more specifics," or "Without knowing more about the job, it's hard for me to answer that." Be honest. Lies will come back to haunt you.

• *It's okay to be nervous.* Don't worry about feeling a little anxious or ticcing more than usual because of the stress. Chances are the interviewer may be somewhat nervous as well, knowing that he or she also is being judged. You can admit to it, then go on with the interview. Don't obsess about being nervous or let anxiety get in your way.

• *It's okay to praise yourself.* There's nothing wrong with having confidence in your abilities and saying, "Yes, I can handle those responsibilities."

• *If you don't get the job, don't automatically figure it is because you have Tourette Syndrome.* (Although it's illegal to disqualify someone because of disabilities, in reality, it does happen.)

There's nothing wrong with calling the person who interviewed you to ask for suggestions for the next time you have an interview. Most people are impressed with someone who wants to improve. The answer may be as simple as "We found someone who knew our particular word-processing program. Otherwise you would have been perfect," or "The woman we hired had more experience." Don't assume the worst. Always strive to do better the next time.

• *Always write a thank-you note after an interview.* You may not have gotten that particular job, but the person you met with may become an important ally. Most jobs are gotten through word-of-mouth, so a previous interviewer may be the one to pass your name along to someone who is hiring.

Write a thank-you letter on business-looking stationery, not notebook paper or pink sheets with flowers or cute kittens. A quick-print shop can help you design proper but inexpensive business stationery with your name, address, and phone number on it or you can ask a friend to compose a letterhead on a computer.

There are many books available that explain how to write a good resume, prepare for an interview, handle an interview, and what you should do to follow-up. Check your local library or bookstore.

CHAPTER 22

Working with Clients and Coworkers

It's likely that you spend more of your waking hours interacting with coworkers than you do with family members, other than on weekends and holidays. Therefore, it seems good common sense to do everything you can to maintain harmony with your "family away from home," those in your place of work.

Most people, if they have Tourette Syndrome or not, have annoying little habits of which they often are totally unaware that can drive their coworkers absolutely crazy. Smoking used to be one such practice, but today it often is not permitted inside offices, hospitals, factories, and other places of work. I used to chew bubble gum while I wrote, cracking and popping it to my heart's content. That was fine when I worked out of my home. No one was around to hear me. Now I have an office in my husband's place of business and have (reluctantly) given up chomping out of courtesy to those near me.

You probably have experienced other work irritators such as the pencil tapper, the person who hums or mumbles to herself, the guy who always uses the speaker phone and shouts into it, the paper crumbler, and the file drawer slammer. This is the chaotic work scene that you, the new employee, enter, adding to the discord of this environment your personal variety of tics—sniffing, hooting, barking, clearing your throat . . . well, you get the idea. Just as the odds are good that at least one person will eventually blow up at the hummer, it's very likely that at some point one of your coworkers is going to tell you just how disturbing your tics are to the others. Why not head off that probable confrontation by telling those at work about your TS? Letting them know that you have Tourette Syndrome often clears the air and explains your behavior before anyone has a chance to judge, belittle, or complain to others about you.

It gives you a chance to educate others about your disorder, which should make your coworkers more understanding and supportive about your symptoms. It also might help them to identify others who have TS and don't know what is wrong with them.

The same is true for your clients. If you feel they may be put off or fearful of your tics, a simple explanation should be reassuring. If they seem interested and ask for additional information, then offer it. If you're good at what you do—and you probably wouldn't have gotten the job if you weren't—then your clients, customers, or patients will accept you for you, and consider your tics merely an impediment, distraction, or inconvenience, like another's stuttering, hearing aid, or cane.

In the final analysis, only you can decide whether or not to tell your coworkers that you have TS. Many people who can hide their symptoms successfully choose not to tell. Those who also have OCD often have concealed their condition from their families and see no reason to do otherwise on the job, although their coworkers might soon notice some of their compulsive behavior.

The following describes how to discuss a disability with employers. Adapted from a brochure dealing with arthritis, the points are equally valid for individuals with TS, ADHD, and OCD.

If you should decide to disclose your disability, plan carefully how and when to discuss the subject with your coworkers or supervisors. Research carefully all the changes that could be made to make your work as productive as possible. Schedule a meeting with your supervisor at a time when neither of you is under pressure. Find an opportunity to talk informally with your coworkers or a personnel officer about ways to make things go more smoothly. In meetings, describe as simply as possible the ways TS (and, if applicable, OCD and ADHD) may affect your work. Make it plain that you are not looking for sympathy, but for ways to resolve the problem that will benefit both the company (or your coworkers) and yourself. The goal of these meetings should be to generate a supportive atmosphere in which everyone works together as part of a team.

Be prepared to help the employer. You are the expert on TS and also on what you need to work efficiently. Offer suggestions for changes that could be made, based on the research you have done before the meeting. Chances are any changes you may need will not cost much. It's a good idea to be as well informed as possible about the ADA, assistive devices you may require and their cost, and resources to help employers. In fact, there may be tax deductions and/or accommodations and/or tax credits available to certain employers who provide accommodations and/or jobs for people with disabilities.[1]

A woman who has worked as a court stenographer for five years admitted that she's never told her employers about her Tourette Syndrome. "I'm very good at masking the symptoms," she said. "When I need to express them, I head for the nearest bathroom. I know the location of every ladies' restroom in the city."

Suppression and substitution of symptoms were used by many employees who had not told anyone at work that they had TS. "They think I have frequent colds because I sniff a lot," said a newspaper reporter.

"I've learned to work the tics I can't suppress into overt gestures," said another. "My coworkers tease that I wouldn't be able to talk with my hands tied behind my back. Little do they know what that kind of restriction would trigger. My tics would drive them from the office."

A surgeon, with numerous motor and vocal tics, said that he had gone all through medical school successfully masking his tics. "They knew I was a little nervous and hyper," he admitted, "but if I had ever told them that I had TS, they would have made

---

[1] Adapted with permission from *Arthritis on the Job: You Can Work with It*, copyright 1994, by the Arthritis Foundation. For further information or for a complete copy of this booklet, write the Arthritis Foundation, P.O. Box 19000, Atlanta, GA 30326, or contact your local Arthritis Foundation chapter.

me go into pathology instead of surgery.'' Fortunately, he is able
to totally suppress tics in the operating room.

Tips for Promoting On-the-Job Harmony

• *Avoid getting overfatigued.* Extreme fatigue can wear down
the strongest among us, lowering the immune system, triggering
emotional extremes, and for those with TS, causing the frequency
and intensity of tics to increase. Even the military learned long
ago that troops who were properly rested held up better in
training. Numerous world figures such as Sir Winston Churchill,
Eleanor Roosevelt, John F. Kennedy, and Thomas Edison found
that a brief catnap refreshed them and allowed them to accomplish
more without feeling fatigued.

Many people with TS report sleep disturbances, either having
difficulty getting to sleep, having restless sleep, or waking early.
Be aware that a good night's sleep can improve on-the-job
harmony considerably. By establishing and maintaining a regular
sleep schedule so you come to work rested, you'll become more
efficient and effective, and better able to focus on the task at
hand.

Limit your overtime work as well. While it may earn you extra
money, the ensuing fatigue also increases tics for most people.
You may also find it more difficult to control your temper when
you're overtired and stressed.

If you also have ADHD, being overtired may cause you to
spend longer than normal on specific tasks and make more
mistakes as you're doing them. Be especially careful if you're
handling money, engaging in work potentially dangerous either
to yourself or others, or utilizing fine motor skills or extreme
concentration.

Become aware of your body/mind condition. Learn to take
catnaps during your coffee break or lunch hour. Practice deep
breathing and other relaxation techniques to refresh yourself. If
you're feeling extremely overtired—physically or mentally—
take advantage of a personal day or half of one if your company's
policy permits it. If you don't enjoy this benefit, make every
effort to try to relax over the weekend.

• *Be positive.* Even if you've found the perfect job, there may be times when you feel overwhelmed and frustrated. Anxiety kicks in, which makes your tics—even those previously responding to medication or actually diminished in frequency and intensity—return. You're angry, feeling threatened by your disorder, your coworkers, and your boss. The cloud of negativity hangs over your head.

That's the time to unleash the power of the mind/body connection. Unfortunately, this is said so often that the true significance of the message often is lost, but it's a fact revealed through scientific studies: when you think positively, your body reacts in a more healthy manner. Your stress level drops, your mind clears, your tics return to their "normal" state, and you can begin to accomplish what needs to be done in order of priorities.

But many of us talk ourselves into failure, limiting our opportunities for success because we tell our body and mind that what we hope to achieve is impossible, that we can never fulfill our dreams.

Become more aware of what you say and think. Are your thoughts and speech filled with negative words such as "I can't," rather than "I can?" "Impossible" rather than "Possible"? In his book, *The Positive Principle Today,* Dr. Norman Vincent Peale wrote, "Of all destructive words in common use, surely one of the most powerful is the word *impossible*. More people have failed by using that one word than almost any other in the English language."

Words do hold meaning and can affect behavior, often adversely. We can develop a more possible attitude toward life and our abilities by consciously selecting positive words and practicing them frequently until they become second nature. Some people call these upbeat words affirmations, while others refer to them as positive self-talk. The meaning is the same, however.

Read some of the anecdotes in the "Success Stories" section of this book and you'll find a number of people who decided that TS was not going to dictate what they could or couldn't do. They succeeded in their personal and professional lives because they intentionally replaced negative thoughts and speech with positive, motivational messages to themselves, and transformed these into positive action. In 1759, English writer Samuel Johnson, who reportedly had both Tourette Syndrome and OCD, wrote that "few things are impossible to diligence and skill."

In their book, *Mind Power,* authors Bernie Zilbergeld, Ph.D., and Arnold A. Lazarus, Ph.D., suggest that by remembering and focusing on past successes, we also can "recreate the feelings of confidence, power, and accomplishment . . . and that helps to ensure good feelings and positive results in the present and future. Recollection of past achievements," they say, "is one of the most powerful kinds of imagery available to anyone."

We all have the power to change, to begin to think positive thoughts and give ourselves upbeat messages that make us believe in ourselves and our ability to accomplish wonders. Often it begins with reeducation, substituting positive words and thoughts for the negative ones. As you can't think of two things at once, thinking positive words and thoughts will leave no room for the negative ones. You'll soon discover that an optimistic approach in your work—regardless if you're a bus driver, teacher, house painter, or social worker—will not only help you to feel more secure and capable in what you do but will make others around you shine in the reflected air of your confidence.

• *Keep a sense of humor.* Some of your coworkers may be insensitive, making little digs or offhand comments about you and/or your tics. Rather than getting angry, try to ignore them or gently make fun of their thoughtlessness.

A little humor can go a long way in defusing situations that may otherwise get out of hand. You can't change how others feel or react to you, but a sense of humor can make *you* feel better, which in the long run may help those taunting you to lighten up a little as well. It also should encourage others to come to your aid.

• *Ask for feedback.* It's hard for us to see ourselves as others do. That's why asking someone whose opinion you respect for constructive feedback can be helpful. You may not always like what you hear, but don't get mad at the person offering the feedback.

Take what you hear seriously. If part of it is negative, ask what you can do to make it more positive. Think in terms of concrete solutions, then do your best to effect a change. Some of the negatives may be due to symptoms of TS, ADHD, and OCD, such as lack of focus, impulsivity, or distractibility, or because of medications you're taking. Acknowledge that influence, but still show a willingness to try to make some changes in order to compensate for your difficulties. Be open to suggestions. If others see you making an effort, usually they'll offer help as well.

If you find yourself bogged down with numerous on-the-job problems and seemingly no solutions, ask for help from a qualified counselor or psychologist, someone who is familiar with work problems related to TS.

• *Check your temper temperature.* Some people with TS find it difficult to keep their anger in check. A mother of a grown son with Tourette Syndrome described three positions her son had lost solely because of his unchecked rages. "At one job, he flew off the handle and started screaming at his coworkers for what he considered to be their lack of motivation and support," she said. "They were dumbfounded. It was like he suddenly exploded without warning. At the second job, I think he just panicked. He felt he couldn't live up to the expectation his superior had for him. As his frustration and perceived loss of confidence by his boss accelerated, he began to throw temper tantrums. He blew up at his staff and even cleared one desktop with a swipe of his hand. It was too bad. He really liked that job. He was fired from the last job for losing his temper with his boss. He just bluntly told him off.

"I used to think it was just boredom, but now I wonder if it's just part of the TS. He's had jobs where one day he just stops going to work. It's not that he doesn't have friends. He's fine socially, but work just seems to be too much pressure. When it builds up, he explodes. He's not able to head it off."

If temper tantrums or attacks of rage have created problems for you at work in the past, try to recall what led up to them and how you felt immediately beforehand. Just as there is a premonitory sensory urge as a tic builds and demands expression, there often are subtle cues before rage attacks develop. If you can become more attuned to these cues, you can either substitute more acceptable behavior or actually remove yourself from situations that are destructive to you, your effectiveness on the job, and your interpersonal relations with those who report to you, your coworkers, and your employers.

CHAPTER 23

Selecting Your Housing

For some adults with Tourette Syndrome, the selection of where to live is easy. As they have no job, they also have no income. Therefore, home is with Mom and Dad. Staying put seems to be the perfect answer for them. It's safe, comfortable, cheap, and the food's good. Why would they want to leave? What's more, sometimes their parents subtly encourage such a situation.

Many parents feel hesitant to shoo young adults from the nest. They've endured so much rejection growing up with TS. We feel that we need to be supportive. We don't want our grown child to think we're tossing him or her out. So other than making subtle (or not-so-subtle) hints, we say nothing.

For some parents, this reluctance to encourage their young adult to leave home is based on need—their own need. "I quit my job to be here for my daughter," a mother admitted. "If she moves out, what do I do?"

Yet, having your own home is an important—albeit somewhat scary—part of becoming an adult. It allows young adults to gain a sense of independence as they leave the family home and go off to create a new home base.

Can Parents Help?

How can parents help their adult children? It really should begin in childhood, as soon as the diagnosis of Tourette Syndrome is made. Parents and other adults in the child's world must ignore the natural (and normal) inclination to surround and protect their youngster from the harshness and expectations of the world. By closing ranks and making the child feel that home is the only place where he or she is truly safe among those who love and understand, we prevent that young person from developing courage and self-confidence. The message we give is that "you are weak and ill-equipped to exist outside this fortress we've created for you." Rather than protecting, however, we will have built a prison and sentenced our child—out of well-meaning love—to a life term of loneliness.

As James Kenneth Whitt, a pediatric psychologist at the University of North Carolina at Chapel Hill described it, "Feelings of vulnerability and inadequacy may become self-fulfilling if, paradoxically, the child withdraws from developmental contention and sustains (or even provokes) interpersonal rejection in order to maintain the now internalized identity as a vulnerable, crippled, socially abandoned person who must depend on close family members for needed care."[1]

Until recently, little had been written or even discussed about the importance of young adults with TS being encouraged to venture out into the world to seek shelter on their own. It wasn't until 1989 that the Tourette Syndrome Association noticed a prevailing theme that kept cropping up at their national conferences: that of providing more services focusing on the day-to-day needs, such as housing, for adults with TS.

"More has been written about fostering independence in young people with diabetes than with TS," Dr. Whitt admitted. "Parents need to be comforted. They know that unlike diabetes or many other chronic disorders, Tourette Syndrome is very visible and the world is a dangerous place. They don't want their child to be exposed. A common response is to become more protective."

One way in which parents can become more reassured about their adult child going out on his or her own is to have what Dr. Whitt calls practice sessions. You probably used this technique

---

[1] Whitt, James Kenneth, "Children's Adaptation to Chronic Illness and Handicapping Conditions," *Chronic Illness and Disability Through the Life Span,* Springer Publishing Company, New York, 1984.

when your child was little and you asked, "What would you do if a stranger asked you to come over to his car?" or "What would you do if I hurt myself and you had to call for help?"

Now that your child is grown and about to go out on his or her own, the practice sessions should center more along the lines of questions like, "How will you explain your tics to a prospective landlord?" or "How will you handle stares or answer questions by other tenants or neighbors?" Hopefully, the responses should give you a comfort zone enabling you to be supportive of your adult child's decision to move out. Role-playing, with you as the landlord or nosey neighbor, can also make your grown child more confident in handling those types of situations.

What Type of Housing Is Best?

Obviously, the best type of housing for someone with TS who has loud vocal tics is one with good soundproofing. That limits the choices considerably since few homes, apartments, condos, or townhouses have adequate soundproofing. In all but single-family homes, you usually can hear toilets flushing, showers running, footsteps clomping, the stereo blasting, and kids crying. In some apartments, you can actually hear your neighbor talking on the telephone or snoring. Therefore, it's very likely that anyone with loud vocal tics will be overheard by his or her neighbors.

If you've ever heard a barking dog next door, a neighbor's kid with a set of drums, or tried to ignore a car alarm going off, you know firsthand that noise pollution can raise blood pressure, make people tense and impatient, and trigger aggression. Studies show that unpredictable noise can become so stressful that, in some cases, people have lost their tempers, attacking and physically injuring those creating the noise. There's no doubt that noise can strain relations between individuals, cause people to be less tolerant of frustration, and make them less willing to help others.

In their booklet, "Guide to Housing for Adults with Tourette Syndrome," the TSA suggests selecting housing in a neighborhood that is partially commercial, so that traffic sounds from the street protect your neighbors from hearing your vocal tics, as well as choosing an apartment with as few common walls as possible, such as an end or corner unit. Consider making your bedroom the one with a common wall since you're less likely to have loud tics at night and your bedroom will buffer sounds you make from the living areas. Carpeting, drapery, wallcovering, and upholstered furniture all help to absorb sound as well.

Check for noise leaks, too. Many walls, especially party walls separating apartment units, are particularly vulnerable to noise leakage. The installation of back-to-back electrical outlets, medicine cabinets, and master cable and television outlets are common causes of noise transference. Inferior construction may have left noninsulated and poorly sealed openings behind cabinets, kitchen appliances, ducts and ventilation grilles, and in closets.

If you have a townhouse or a home on a zero lot line, your concerns with sound may be lessened. Nevertheless, as your neighbors may still be in close proximity, consider buying an air-conditioning unit so you can keep your windows closed. Meet with your neighbors so they'll understand what's happening if they hear your vocalizations while you're sunbathing or grilling outdoors.

Do what you can to "sound soften" your living quarters, then relax. Home should be the one place you don't have to think about withholding your tics, and with some preplanning, it's possible.

The TSA publication "Guide to Housing for Adults with Tourette Syndrome" also contains specific information on Fair Housing Laws, types of housing, advice on obtaining legal counsel, and tips on how to help bolster soundproofing.

How to Handle Neighbors

Unless you pitch a tent in the middle of a desert, on an isolated island, or on a ranch with nothing nearby but cattle and cactus, you probably *will* have neighbors. They may be down at the next farm or on the next block, but you'll see them jogging, as you're getting your mail, and taking out the trash. While you can figure, "To heck with them. I have as much right to live here as they do" (and you'd be right), it's easier to get along with neighbors. You never know when you might need to borrow some milk or need their phone to report that yours is out. This is especially important for those with ADHD who may blow up at others without thinking of the consequences.

If your symptoms are such that they're bound to be noticed— medium to severe verbal and motor tics—consider telling your neighbors about TS, either face-to-face or in writing. If they don't know what's wrong and you just glare when they stare, they may be afraid, thinking you're weird or dangerous. This is a violent world today, and anyone who's "different" is suspect. If you've just moved into an apartment or condo, send a letter to your neighbors describing TS in general and your tics in particular. That way they won't send for the police when they hear shrieks or shouting coming from your unit or run out of the laundry room when they see you coming. Remember, we're all afraid of the unknown.

As long as you're in the educating mode, remember that a change of address will probably also mean changing many of the businesses with whom you have previously dealt. You'll need to reeducate bank officials in your new branch, the hair stylist, employees at the grocery, health club, and so on.

Don't make a big production out of this revelation. Just introduce yourself, say that you've moved into the neighborhood, plan to frequent their business establishment, and that you have Tourette Syndrome, a neurological disorder that causes verbal and motor tics. Hand them the "Q & A" pamphlet printed by the TSA or an information sheet that you have created. By talking to them calmly and unemotionally, you give the nonverbal message that you are "okay," in control (even though you cannot control your tics), and a potential valued customer.

A new home base also may mean taking a different bus or public transportation to work. If you have noticeable tics, especially coprolalia, you may need to explain to those around you. One young man was ordered off his new bus the first day for "talking dirty." He gave the bus driver a card he had created with information about TS. Now the driver is his best publicist and helps to educate others along that route. If your coprolalia includes the shouting of racial or ethnic slurs, travel on public transportation during off-peak hours whenever possible for your own safety. Someone may hit (or shoot) before you can tell him or her about TS.

CHAPTER 24

Celebrating Success Stories

You may be reading this book while still in shock, just having received the diagnosis that your child—or perhaps you yourself—has TS, a chronic disorder that is, at this writing, incurable.

One woman interviewed for this book was an adult when she finally learned she had not only Tourette Syndrome but also OCD. "I always sensed there was really something wrong," she said. "I didn't *feel* crazy. So, I made the best of what I had. I'm glad I didn't wait for a diagnosis before starting to enjoy life."

Another, who also was diagnosed in adulthood, said, "When you have Tourette Syndrome as badly as I've had, you only have two choices: One, I could become a recluse, or two, I could overcompensate for my problems and become somebody. I chose the latter and I've never been sorry." She is now a junior high school teacher and a TS advocate.

Below are the stories of many people—youngsters as well as adults—who decided to turn the lemons of TS in their lives into lemonade. Among them you'll find a surgeon, lawyer, physicist, educator, soldier, sports figures—in short, people in many professions who have successfully accommodated the symptoms of Tourette Syndrome into their everyday lives.

Some of these individuals describe symptoms that have not been proven by research as being part of the definition of TS. Nevertheless, as they are experienced by these people and others, I've included those characteristics in the following stories.

Susan Conners

I met Susan at the 1993 National Conference on Tourette Syndrome in Houston. She not only was a speaker at one of the break-out sessions but she also was the National Conference chairperson. Susan was diagnosed with TS in her late thirties after seeing it portrayed on the *Quincy* television show. She first displayed symptoms of the disorder when she was six years old. In second or third grade, she also developed symptoms of OCD, especially expressing counting and erasing compulsions.

"I grew up on a farm and went to a one-room school," she said. "In retrospect, I feel sorry for the teacher. There were seventeen kids. Four were my siblings and we all had Tourette Syndrome. She never said anything about our noises and motor tics. I guess she just thought we were like our mother. She had TS too."

Because Susan Conners didn't know what was wrong with her—and because her siblings all had similar vocal and motor tics—she never considered herself handicapped, and grew up assuming that she could do anything. Zeroing in on the teaching profession, she received her undergraduate degree in education, and earned a master's degree at the University of Buffalo.

"Interviewing for my student teaching assignment was a nightmare," she recalled. "Because no one knew what caused my symptoms, everyone assumed I was just a nervous person. I had eye blinks, jerking arms, and kept throwing my head back. Nevertheless, I got a student teaching job, where I still teach French to eighth graders. I felt I had to be an overachiever to prove myself worthy of that trust.

"The students in my classroom are terrific," she said. "They ask about my tics and we talk openly about them. I welcome the opportunity to educate people about TS. Right now there are four kids in the building with Tourette Syndrome. I gave an in-service so all the teachers and students would understand what was going on. Afterwards, one of my kids came up to me and said, 'You're the bravest person I know.'

"It still causes me pain when I'm asked to leave a movie. Usually I'll explain about TS to the usher and sit in the back so

I can dash out if I need to. On airplanes I sit by the window so I won't bother others with my tics. I work at holding the tics in and sometimes it's exhausting. When they're finally expressed, they're more severe than they would have normally been.

"My advice to others? Be accepting of yourself. My friends say they don't notice my tics anymore. They're just part of the way I am. Also, keep a sense of humor. It helps others to feel more comfortable and makes you feel better too.

"We had a new teacher who didn't know me. When she saw my hands flying around in the lunchroom, she asked innocently, 'Do you teach sign language?' Everyone froze, waiting to see my reaction. I laughed and said, 'Can you imagine how confused a kid would be if I signed this way?' We all laughed together. I made a friend of the new teacher because I helped her cover her embarrassment.

"I see a lot of bitter people with Tourette Syndrome. What a waste. Although I wouldn't have asked for it, TS has served me well. It's given me great rapport with my students. I also work with a TS youth support group. I have the kids tell the others one sad thing and one funny thing that has happed to them since our last meeting. It helps them get in touch with their emotions. Laughter and tears. We need them both."

Jim Eisenreich[1]

If you're a baseball fan, you've heard of Jim Eisenreich, right fielder for the Philadelphia Phillies, outstanding defensive player, and a super slugger. For much of the first half of the 1993 season, he either led the team or was second in batting average. After midseason, Jim was batting an incredible .330, heading toward his best season ever in the major leagues (he had hit a grand slam home run and was on a pace to set career records for himself in several categories). In fact, in 1993, the Phillies won the National

---

[1] Adapted from articles written by Alan Levitt and used by permission of both Alan Levitt and the Tourette Syndrome Association.

League pennant and Jim hit a home run in the World Series. Not bad for someone who, in his rookie year with the Minnesota Twins in 1982, was admitted to a psychiatric hospital because he twitched, grunted, and snorted.

Yes, Jim Eisenreich has Tourette Syndrome. But although he'd had involuntary movements and vocalizations since he was six, he didn't know what was wrong until he was diagnosed during the 1984–85 season. Even then, the team physician for the Minnesota Twins doubted the diagnosis, incorrectly thinking you had to have coprolalia in order to have TS.

Today Jim serves as a role model for young people with Tourette Syndrome. A spiritual man, he senses the importance of his impact on others struggling to cope with the symptoms of TS and works toward increasing public awareness and understanding of the disorder. He took part in a panel discussion at the 1991 TSA National Conference in Washington, D.C., organizes TSA Bowl-a-Thons, speaks about TS at schools, and arranges for youngsters with TS to come to his baseball games.

Jim is married to the former Leann Danner. They have a son and a daughter. When asked if he worried about his children having TS, he shook his head. "God never gives us more than we can handle."

Mort Doran, M.D., M.Sc., F.R.C.S.

Mort Doran is a Canadian general surgeon who also happens to have Tourette Syndrome along with OCD. While it sounds like an impossible marriage of profession and disorders, Doran is just one of a number of surgeons who have Tourette Syndrome. He didn't learn what he had until he was long out of medical school, thirty-six years old, and a practicing surgeon. A neurologist on the radio was describing the symptoms of TS and, for the first time, Doran heard the words *Tourette Syndrome*.

"I knew immediately that he was talking about me. I was seven when I started having tics," he recalled, "but my behavior problems preceded those by years. Everyone said I was a 'bitchy' kid. When I was three I remember kicking an aunt for no particular reason. I also remember being literally dragged down to the principal's office when I was in kindergarten, so I must have done something pretty awful. As with many people, my behavioral disorder caused more problems than my tics.

"I think my first tic was blinking. My parents said, 'Don't do that anymore.' So I didn't. I began nodding my head instead. When they said 'Stop it!' I began to move it side to side. For a while the tics remained in my upper body, settling for a while on my shoulders. If I tightened one, I had to tighten the other. My parents, who had adopted me when they were in their forties, used to say, 'How can you do this to us? We picked you out of the lineup. We chose you over the others.' Did I feel guilty!"

Talking to me in a Chicago apartment, where he had come to speak before both medical and lay groups, Dr. Doran spoke openly about his life with TS. His vocal pattern was reminiscent of Robin Williams; his body was in constant motion. Like many men who have facial hair, he constantly played with and plucked at the hairs of his beard and mustache, but he also mumbled "bald . . . bald" under his breath. He tugged at first one sleeve, then the other. "Supersensitive. The material makes my skin feel . . . strange."

Dr. Doran continued to pull at his sleeves. "If I touch one, I have to touch the other, to even it up." He tapped the table and glanced, so I thought, at his watch. He caught my expression. "No, no. I'm not looking at my watch. We've all day to talk. It's just one of my tics. If you were closer, I'd tap your head or shoulders. I do that too." He spoke calmly, even jokingly. I was impressed with his comfort level. Before too much longer, I no longer noticed his tic routine.

"Noises bothered me too," he continued. "If my mother clanked the dishes after dinner while she was washing up, I couldn't study. All extraneous noises bothered me. I couldn't stand my father's chomping or slurping his soup at mealtime, so I had to eat apart from him. I just was supersensitive to sound too. Everything had to be silent. Now it doesn't seem to bother me. In fact, I usually have background music playing while I read.

"Reading, however, was and still is difficult for me. I hated

English class," he said, shaking his head either at the memory or as a tic. "I had to center everything in my field of vision so it was perfectly symmetrical. I counted letters, repeated words over and over again. I kept going back to reread what I had just read. Obviously, I read very slowly. I still have difficulty with reading, and to this day, I don't read novels. I'm just too distractible. On the other hand, I do stay current with my medical journals. It's slow, arduous work, and takes me longer than most people. Medical school was hard only because of all the reading. I read everything so painstakingly that eventually I had it memorized.

"As a kid, I got teased a lot because of my tics. I stayed pretty much on my own so I didn't have to answer to anyone. We lived next to a ravine. I'd take some sandwiches and books there and spend the whole day in the ravine. I also got into walking, which I still enjoy. In high school, I both wanted to belong and I didn't. I got into a high school fraternity, but they had me do stupid things as a pledge. My behavioral problems made it difficult for me to take orders, so I eventually quit."

After graduating from the University of Toronto, Doran decided to go to medical school. In 1957, no interview was necessary, so he just filled out a questionnaire on "Why Do You Want to Be a Doctor?" and was accepted.

"Perhaps if I had known that I had TS and OCD I wouldn't have attempted medical school," he mused, "so it was probably just as well I didn't know. If *they* had known what I had, they probably would never have let me become a surgeon. I would have ended up in pathology. But I was fairly successful at suppressing my tics so they just figured I was a little nervous. Sometimes they'd ask, 'Are you cold?' because it looked as though I was shivering.

"I hated being talked down to while I was in medical school, but I knew I'd have to accept it if I wanted to become a doctor. The same was true of all the dumb things you have to do over and over again while you're a medical student and a resident. I wanted to talk back, but held it in. It wasn't easy. My residency was done with great difficulty because I came so close so many times to exploding. But I'd mentally compute the damages and knew it wasn't worth being thrown out. Perhaps if I'd known what was wrong with me I could have defused the situation. As it was, I didn't have an option, so I went along with the program.

"I still have temper outbursts that are uncontrollable. It was very distressing for my two sons (now teenagers) when they were young. They couldn't understand why it was okay for me to throw the fruit bowl off the table or kick the wall and they couldn't. My wife taught them to follow her lead and just walk away. The rage storm usually ends quickly and I'm fine, other than feeling very foolish that I couldn't control my impulses better. It's as though my impulse circuits are plugged in wrong. I seem to have the temper control of a two-year-old. We both throw tantrums, but while the toddler doesn't care, I'm embarrassed.

"When I get angry, it's usually totally out of proportion with the incident that triggered it. A bicycler once shouted at me when I made a left turn in front of him. I erupted, hitting my steering wheel and fantasizing going back and running him over with the car until he was dust. For years, whenever I came to the four-way stop where the incident occurred, I ruminated over it. I'm not a violent man; I'd never hit another person. Yet I was furious at this unknown biker.

"I've never lost my temper in the operating room and I've never had any tics that interfered with my surgical technique. It isn't that I've stifled the impulses; they've just never happened and I'm comfortable that they never will. It just shows how selective these things are."

Dr. Doran has been on Prozac for the last two years. Although it does not diminish the tics in any way, it lessens his rage impulses considerably. "I still skip when I walk and tap parking meters and cars, but thanks to Prozac, I don't lash out or grit my teeth holding back my temper when faced with customs agents and police the way I used to."

Dr. Doran is adopted and expresses great interest in those with TS who also were adopted as children. "There's no question that there is a higher percentage of adopted kids with TS than one would think. It may be that there is something that triggers a genetic disposition to TS. Maybe it's being in an orphanage as I was or perhaps maternal stress during pregnancy triggers it. Researchers are looking into the adoption issues.''

What advice does Dr. Doran have for others? ''Don't use your TS as an excuse. It's a reason why you do things, not an excuse for why you can't.

''Whatever you do, do something where you can be your own boss. Most people with TS have low tolerance levels for being subservient and not in command. Open up your own corner store, if necessary, or become a business consultant. It doesn't matter if you sweep the floor or tell others to. You're the boss.

''Probably the most important advice I can offer is to learn to take responsibility for yourself. If you're the parent of a child with TS, teach your youngster this. We have to learn to live within the structure of our world. We can make adaptations, so it's easier for us to adjust, but we can't make excuses.

''Tics are really not such a big deal. Oh, I know it's easy to talk that way from where I am now. It hurt as a youngster. I got teased about my tics when I was in school, but then I also got teased about wearing glasses and having bands on my teeth. But people, especially as you get older, can see past the tics. It's the antisocial behavior that others won't tolerate.

''Teach your children to learn to substitute more acceptable behavior for their impulsive antisocial responses. For example, if they have the urge to touch a woman's breasts, suggest that they redirect their actions by asking if they can pat the head or shoulders instead. Let them hit a punching bag instead of their sister or go outside at school and throw bean bags rather than books in the classroom.

''Set limits and rules for kids with TS. These may be different than those you set for his or her siblings, but there must be limits. Tell them, 'You can bang on the countertop, but you can't throw dishes.' As for hitting or hurting others, that's never negotiable.

''You can do about anything you want, although I don't think I'd go to an auction. With my tics I'd look as though I was bidding on everything. But aside from that, even with TS I have had a long and successful surgical practice, I've had my private pilot operator's license since 1967, and I'm married and have two teenage sons who are extremely dear to me.

"You need to keep your perspective. As a physician, I've seen so many terrible diseases and what they can do. I'd rather have TS than a lot of other worse things."

Dr. Doran was keynote speaker at the 1993 Tourette Syndrome Conference in Houston. He concluded his remarks by saying, "I walked up here to get to the podium, and some people can't walk; I'm speaking to all of you, and some cannot talk; I look out in the audience and see all of you, and others can't see. All in all, I'd say I'm pretty lucky."

Lauren Liona

If you talked on the telephone to fourteen-year-old Lauren Liona, you'd be impressed with her verbal skills, sense of humor, and unusual maturity and poise for her age. Along with those outstanding qualities, Lauren also has a severe case of Tourette Syndrome including self-injurious behavior (at age six she cut herself on the belly with a knife), coprolalia, echolalia, and copropraxia. She also has ADHD and OCD.

"My earliest memory is of being two," she said. "I scrunched up my face. My parents thought I was just being cute. I felt confused because I didn't know why I was doing it." Quickly she ran through her past history, anxious to talk about the present. "In kindergarten, I couldn't sit still. I was always being put in the corner. In first grade, I started snorting. My mother thought it was my adenoids, but it wasn't. In second grade, I got punishment assignments, which meant having to write 'I won't make noises' thirty times. It was hard. I knew I couldn't stop making that noise. Third grade was great."

"Why?" I asked.

"The teacher loved me," she said. "I was cherished." Then she reflected, "I was class president that year. I had friends. A good year. I started doing strange movements then . . . I'd swoop down, hop, then touch the ground. But I made excuses."

She was silent, remembering that wonderful third-grade year. "What happened in fourth grade?" I prompted.

"It was awful. I started tapping on the desk with my pen or

pencil. I had obsessions about taking a knife and cutting the teacher. She made my life a living hell. She told the class to make fun of me so I'd stop tapping and making noises. For punishment, I had to wash all thirty of the desks. That was when I was diagnosed with Tourette Syndrome. It was tough on a little girl. A heavy load. I was happy because I finally knew it wasn't just a bad habit, but I was sad because I began to understand what I'd be facing.

"The teacher thought my mother saying I had Tourette Syndrome was just making an excuse for what I did. My fifth grade was no better. That teacher really was blown away by my tics. She treated me like a 'retard.' She held class discussions about me in front of me, like I couldn't understand.

"Sixth grade was junior high school. Things got really bad. I blinked a lot then. Someone shoved me against a wall and said, 'Stop blinking.' I said I couldn't help it. So he took a knife out of his pocket and cut me on my chin. I still have the scar.

"The kids in junior high would circle me in the hallway and yell at me, calling me 'freak.' There was a large group of kids in my neighborhood who also took delight in tormenting me. They'd throw rocks and call me 'troll' or 'demon.'

"For seventh grade, I got to go to a private school. It's for kids with ADHD, OCD, or other disabilities. The classes are small, twelve or thirteen kids. We talk about not making fun of others because all of us have something.

"I have coprolalia too. Before the diagnosis, my mother washed my mouth out with soap because I embarrassed her. My father punished me too. I don't blame them. They didn't know.

"Now my little brother is showing symptoms of TS. I feel badly for my mother. I feel her pain. It makes me feel weird to know he's going to have it too. I know he won't be alone with it like I was. I can help him. I tried to explain about TS in a way he can understand. I said it was like a little bug that goes through a family as far back as you can count. If the little bug wakes up in someone, you have TS.

"I can suppress the tics for a short time, like when my mom is making a message for the telephone answering machine or when I go to the library, although I don't go too often. When we go shopping, I need my mom not to be embarrassed by me. I've developed my own identity. I don't try to fit in or be like other people. I'm not. I have Tourette Syndrome. If someone stares at me because of my tics, I'll either smile at them or tell them I have TS. They're either interested and ask questions or walk away. I figure it's their problem.

"After college, I want to go into zoology. I love animals. I have five tortoises, three birds (one parrot and two parakeets), three hamsters, a rabbit, four toads, and a chicken. I also learn about them.

"Animals replace the emptiness of friends," she answered matter-of-factly. "I don't have friends." Then she paused. "There is one girl who I'm sort of friends with, but her parents don't like her spending too much time with me."

"What about a boyfriend?" I asked.

Lauren giggled like a typical fourteen-year-old girl. "Well . . . I *do* have a boyfriend. He's a real gentleman. I met him at the pool. He doesn't care that I have TS. His older brother is severely retarded. My boyfriend doesn't treat me like I am. He understands the difference.

"I always think about having kids one day," Lauren added. "I wouldn't let my having TS stop me. They'd always know where to turn. I'd always be there for them, like my mom has been for me."

It was apparent that Lauren and her mother are very close. "We have excellent communication," her mother said. "But we don't switch places. She knows I'm the mother and she's the daughter. But we listen to one another. For a long time, I tried to protect Lauren from the world. Now she tells me how much she can take. She dips when she walks. I've learned that if she says she's taking her bike to go half a block, it's because she feels more comfortable riding than being teased about her way of walking.

"We had two years of family therapy with the TS group. I learned that I have the right to get frustrated with her tics—even though I know she can't help them—and that I have the right to tell her how I feel. I strongly recommend family counseling for everyone—parents, siblings, extended family, and the child with

TS. You all have to be fully cognizant of whatever is going on.''

As with many individuals with TS, Lauren doesn't like clothes that fit tightly (like stirrup pants) or wool and will only wear socks without a heel seam. At present she is on medication including Prozac, clonidine (the Catapres patch), and Risperdal. Haldol was ineffective for her and the ensuing fatigue makes her refer to it as "the drug from hell." (NOTE: Others have used Haldol successfully and find the side effects tolerable. Reactions to medications are extremely individual.)

She had plenty of advice for other teenagers with TS:

- Whatever gets in your way, just knock it down.
- Form your own identity. Be yourself; don't strive to be what you aren't.
- Don't care what others think; care about yourself.
- Communicate. Talk about what you have. Don't be afraid to have others walk away, even if it's a really cute boy. If he walks away, he doesn't deserve you.
- Ask for help when you need it.

Mahmoud Abdul-Rauf [2]

Those who watched the 1994 NBA playoffs marveled at the talent of Denver Nugget star, Mahmoud Abdul-Rauf. If he looked somewhat familiar to fans, it's because prior to the summer of 1993, he played under his birth name of Chris Jackson, the same Chris Jackson who left LSU after his sophomore year to enter the NBA draft (he was the No. 3 pick) and was signed by the Denver Nuggets.

During the summer of 1993, he legally changed his name to Mahmoud Abdul-Rauf, which means "praiseworthy, merciful, and kind," to affiliate himself more with the Muslim religion, to which he had converted in 1991.

---

[2] Adapted from articles and other material written by Alan Levitt. Used by permission of Alan Levitt and the Tourette Syndrome Association.

Although the 1991–92 season was disappointing for him and he didn't get much playing time, his 1992–93 season was a spectacular one. Not only did he lead the team in most categories, he was also second in the entire NBA in free-throw accuracy (93.5 percent). He finished that season making 59 straight free-throws. Sportswriters voted him "Most Improved Player" in the NBA for the 1992–93 season.

In the 1994 regular season, Rauf led his team in number of field goals, highest percentage of free-throws, most assists, and overall point average. In the NBA Conference semifinals against the Utah Jazz he scored the most field goals and the most points for his team.

Because of basketball's fast pace and the speed at which television cameras flash from one player to another, many fans may not notice Rauf rolling his shoulders, jerking his head, and blinking when the game's tempo slows momentarily. They don't hear him shouting, "Whoops," or "Uh-huh." Yes, this star player also has Tourette Syndrome. While some newscasters speculated that his medication hurt his play in the 1991–92 season, Rauf is quick to deny that.

"The main difference [in his play] has been God and my attitude," he said. "He gives me strength. I'm more focused. I don't let anything bother me. From now on for the rest of my career no matter where I'm at, I got to be on a mission—that has to be my attitude; go out every night and play hard."

Rauf was seventeen before he was diagnosed with TS. Before then, friends and family just thought he was a little strange with those odd noises, weird jerks and twitches, funny way of repeating what others had just said, and perfectionistic tendencies.

When asked if he had anything specific to say to those with TS, Rauf answered, "God gives you an infirmity, but also he gives you a strength. For me, my weakness may be Tourette, but for my strength, He's given me basketball and the knowledge to understand people—and the ability to understand myself.

"Whether you are a basketball player or an artist, it's up to you to find that strength and deal with it to overcome your weakness.

As long as you keep God, you can persevere through your hard times and stay confident and positive about everything. You can do everything that you want to—that's what I feel.''

Gary Marmer, Ph.D.

Since 1972, Gary James Marmer has been employed as a physicist, working for the Environmental Assessment and Information Sciences Division of the Argonne National Laboratory, which is owned by the Department of Energy and run by the University of Chicago. Author of more than fifty journals, books, reports, and conference publications, Marmer has also served as an expert witness, presenting testimony on cooling systems at six Atomic Safety and Licensing Board hearings. And yes, he has Tourette Syndrome along with ADHD and OCD.

"My tics began when I was five," he recalled in a telephone interview. "I'd spin around and touch the ground. Then, it just went away. Soon afterward, however, I developed an eye blink. The doctor told my parents that I was a nervous child. We never discussed it, not even when I later developed vocal tics such as grunting and clearing my throat.

"I don't remember ever being teased about my tics, other than once when I was in high school and had a summer job surveying with the City of Cincinnati. The other workers ridiculed me. No one else ever did because I got pretty good at hiding them.

"English and history were pretty difficult in high school. I found reading to be hard. My mind started wandering after I had just done a couple of sentences. Even now, I'm restless. I can't stay in my seat for more than five minutes. If I need to talk to my secretary, I'll get up and go to her, rather than buzzing for her.

"Math, on the other hand, was always easy for me. I knew in high school that I wanted to go into physics. I picked my college, Case Institute of Technology (now Case Western), because I had fallen in love at first sight with a girl from Cleveland. She came to a Young Judea conference in Cincinnati and I spotted her when I met the train. We dated all through college and got married when I graduated.

"Despite the fact that I had tics and was compulsive—getting places early because I couldn't stand being late, getting out of the car, locking it, checking, putting the key in my pocket, checking it, or checking every five minutes to be sure I still had the plane tickets when we traveled—she never mentioned anything. I always felt it was something deep and dark in my background, some psychological abnormality, and I think she respected my privacy.

"Stress made my tics much worse. They really got out of hand when I was at Ohio State University in 1968, working on my Ph.D. in physics. That was the only time I felt I needed counseling. It wasn't helpful, though. They told me I was having tics because I wasn't working hard enough.

"It wasn't until I was thirty-nine that I finally learned there was a name for my disorder. The *Chicago Tribune* ran an article about TS. I said, 'That's me!' I called the number they listed for the TSA in Bayside, New York. They referred me to a wonderful woman, Lilly Frandzel, who had a grown son with TS. She was one of the original founders of the Chicago chapter. I immediately became active in it, partly to learn as much as I could about TS and partly to help others. I often go to schools at the request of a parent to talk to the teachers and administrators about TS.

"There have been some strange moments caused by my TS. One of my tics or compulsions is to touch things. I don't touch people, but that's about the only exception. A few years ago I went to Amsterdam and visited their famous art museum, the Rijksmuseum. Predictably, I touched the frame on one of the masterpieces. Immediately, alarms went off and the doors locked. I explained why I had touched the painting and they were very understanding.

"A similar situation occurred at the British Museum in London. There I touched an emergency exit door and I guess I hit it with too much force. Anyway, I set their alarm off too. Like the Dutch, the British officials were most compassionate when I explained my compulsion, even though they had never heard of TS.

"Most of the time, however, I can control my tics in public. I bang my head on the headrest when I get into my car. I do it on airplanes too. I smell things too—my hands mostly—and look at the sun, even though I know I shouldn't. Sometimes I sniff. Every now and then my neck hurts because I've been jerking it. The only medication I've ever been on is clonidine and I started taking that for high blood pressure.

"I really don't make an effort to tell people what I have as it really doesn't interfere that much in my life. I have three grown children, one of whom has a mild case of Tourette Syndrome. My paternal grandmother and two of her sisters had tics, so I guess the genetic considerations do have some basis."

Captain Mike Higgins

"According to my mother," said former U.S. Army Captain Mike Higgins, "I always had tics, although I really don't remember. I certainly had no problem with them at school, although I had ADHD. I learned by *not* paying attention. I just got bored quickly. My arm jerked so my handwriting wasn't too good. I had the head jerks that I still have. It made reading difficult because I kept losing my place.

"I grew up in a tough neighborhood in North St. Louis, a ghetto area of African-Americans. The teachers in my district were so glad you actually showed up for class that they weren't about to send you home because of a few tics."

This soft-spoken officer in his late thirties used this type of self-depreciating humor throughout my interview with him.

"I went through basic training when I was twenty-one," he continued. "The structure of army life was and is perfect for someone as obsessive as I am. The military should love a person with a mild case of TS. My compulsive behavior made me a model officer. I did everything by the book, according to regulation." He never received less than a superior evaluation.

"Of course," he admitted, "I did get frustrated more often than other officers because I tried to fine-tune everything."

He's learned to suppress his tics—head jerking, loud grunting sounds, and echolalia (repeating someone's last few words)—when necessary. "It's like holding your breath all the time. But I could hold the tics back when I briefed generals or when I appeared in public. When I've been on television, I try to control my tics by holding the seam of my trousers.

"The army's where I felt comfortable. It's compatible with my behavior. I was in field artillery for a while. The noises *I* make were minute when compared to the sounds the cannons made. But I don't think I could be a librarian. It's too quiet."

That comment made me ask about his most recent career decision. An ordained minister since 1981, Mike's now studying at the Covenant Seminary School in St. Louis for his master's degree so he can become an army chaplain. "If quiet bothers you, how can you preach in a church?"

"I'm a Baptist," he laughed. "We can get pretty loud. Nobody notices *my* making noises." Then he grew serious. "My TS makes me obsessive when it comes to my preaching. I can't sleep if I don't think I'm well prepared. I'll get up early just to check that I've got the right scripture, then double-check. I'm always checking behind myself. I couldn't sleep if I didn't check."

As with most people with TS, Mike doesn't try to suppress his tics at home. "When I come home, I'm tired. Then my tics are really loud. My daughter was on the phone once, talking to a friend. Her friend said, 'I didn't know you had a dog.' My daughter answered 'That's not a dog. That's my father.'

"I'm obsessive around the house. The first thing I do when I walk in is take out the trash. My wife and two daughters make a game of it. I'm always clearing up. I can't stand clutter. I straighten all the hangers in the closet so they face the same way.

"I also hate bright lights. Always have, even as a kid. They make me feel cold. My mother used to fuss that I read in the dark. I loved blackout conditions in the field. We *had* to use flashlights.

My wife knows to switch off the overhead and turn on the lamps when I'm due home.

"I've always had sleep problems, which seems to be typical for many with TS. Even as a child, my mother said I never took naps. I read myself to sleep, trying to drift off. Often my tics keep me from sleeping. Unfortunately, if I don't get enough sleep, my tics are worse at work."

Mike and his wife, Renee, have been married since 1978. Director of a day-care center and mother of their two teenage daughters, Renee acknowledges that Mike's tics are worse at home because he doesn't have to hold them in. "When we were dating, I noticed that he blinked and cleared his throat a lot," she said. "I thought he had allergies. The more time we spent together, the more I noticed other tics. Although I had heard of Tourette Syndrome, I never thought of it in regard to Mike. TS sounded like some exotic disease. You know, 'Oh, that cursing disease.'

"But I didn't marry Tourette Syndrome. I married Mike. There are gives and takes in every relationship. When his tics and associated behaviors bother me—and they sometimes do—I try to remember that it's not Mike, it's the TS. So I let him take out every trash bag around. We joke about it. It's like a game. And although he doesn't tic when he's sleeping, he does kick me in bed.

"You learn to live with whoever you live with," she added. "I have things Mike doesn't like. I've learned not to do things I know will get him upset. I've learned from him too. His side of the closet is neater than mine; all of his hangers go the same way."

Mike once apologized to a coworker for making disruptive noises. "Don't worry," the fellow officer said. "If you ever stop, I'd think something was wrong."

Mike Higgins has made TS work for him in a positive way. "TS makes you increase your professionalism," he said. "My advice to others is to try to turn a liability into an asset. Parents shouldn't let the fear drive them further than they need to go, like filling their children up with medication trying to make all of the tics go away. I think that's overreacting, being preoccupied with totally eradicating every sign of TS. Nobody overreacted with me so I learned to adjust to TS and go on with making a life for myself. I never let my disorder stand in my way. I've had no medication since 1986 and feel much better for it. The most important thing to remember is that Tourette Syndrome doesn't affect what kind of talent you have.''

James A. "Merk" Merklinger

"I'm six feet two inches tall, white, and have Tourette Syndrome with coprolalia. You can imagine how I stood out from the crowd the year I taught English in Japan.''

This twenty-eight-year-old lawyer has learned to laugh at himself and his tics. "I was five or six when my tics began,'' he told me during a phone interview, his sentences interspersed by coprolalia. "My head jerked and I gnashed my teeth. Doctors told my parents I was a repressed child.

"I played all sports in junior and senior high school. I was a pitcher when I was eleven or twelve and remember having to touch my sternum before each pitch. I had no tics while playing football or reading and set records in six positions in football. Still, I didn't have a lot of self-confidence. When my teammates elected me captain of the team, I thought they were doing it as a joke.

"I was diagnosed when I was fourteen and have three younger siblings with TS. But I've never let it get me down. I tell people, 'I have Tourette Syndrome; it doesn't have me.' I always worked hard and had good rapport with my coaches and teachers. I have amazing friends and a great girlfriend. They just accept the tics, even the coprolalia, as part of me.

"I have tactile sensitivity and hated wearing a tight football uniform. I stopped wearing my hip pads and didn't hook the shoulder pads. That felt better.

"There were times both in college (Fork Union Military Academy, then Wofford College) and in law school (University of South Carolina) that I just couldn't study because of the tics. I'd go work out. I think it helped indirectly. It also helped me to stay in shape.

"I didn't take any medication while I was in college. In law school, I tried taking Orap, but it knocked me out. I decided not to take anything even though the tics were bad then. I was allowed an extra thirty minutes extension on each section of the bar exam and took it in a separate room with a supervisor. There were fifteen of us who received special accommodations for testing. A lot of people don't know that it is available to them. Having nontimed exams helps to reduce the natural stress from a test situation.

"I've served as an altar boy and been in the weddings of several friends and one of my brothers. I don't tic then. My attitude when on stage or giving a speech is that the tics aren't important, the speech is, so I concentrate on the speech and don't notice the tics.

"The TS was worse for me when I didn't know what was wrong or why I was acting so weird. When I was fourteen, I was in the hospital in Washington for tests and got friendly with a nine-year-old girl. She had leukemia and wore a wig because her hair had all fallen out. I felt awful when she died, but her death made me realize that I wasn't going to die from TS. I decided right then that I wouldn't let it stop me. I became more outgoing and tried to be the best all-around person, athlete, scholar, whatever. I'm not the fastest or the smartest, but I was going to be the best me I could be."

Merk's advice to others with TS is:

• Find out all you can about TS so you can tell others.
• Tell others. If it doesn't bother you, it won't bother them.

Joanne E. Cohen

It took a number of attempts before I finally was able to interview Joanne Cohen, a thirty-two-year-old woman with a severe case of Tourette Syndrome. She was having difficulty regulating her medication. She felt "dopey" and her voice was slurred. After almost a month, we spoke by phone.

"I was in fourth grade when I started with an eye blink and a shoulder shrug," she said. My pediatrician said it was a transient tic and sent me to a psychiatrist who I saw three days a week. Finally, when I was thirteen, I was diagnosed as having TS.

"I took Haldol until I went to college. I reacted badly to it, sleeping through eighth grade. I'd get up late for school, sleep through class, go to the nurse's office where I'd sleep, attend Spanish class, then go home and sleep some more. In ninth grade we got it titrated better. I went to a private school and did well despite having mild grunting and squeaks. I graduated top of my class and went to Boston University where I majored in psychology.

"My first semester, I went home for Thanksgiving. I was sitting in the kitchen with my parents when I suddenly said 'shit,' and kept repeating it. My mother thought, 'Oh, no,' but it was the beginning of my coprolalia. My heart sank. I had heard others with it at TS meetings and remember thinking, 'At least I'm not like that.' And now I was.

"At that time I also had a motor tic that made me spin around and I said 'un huh,' all the time. Kids at school called me the 'huh huh bird.' I asked for and got a private room in the dorm, referred to as a 'medical single.'

"I was involved in student government, the honor society for psychology, and the hiking club. I was very active in student life despite my tics, which I couldn't mask. I had a small group of friends and went to hockey games with them, but I was embarrassed to discuss my Tourette Syndrome, which had gotten pretty bad. My tics were loud; sometimes I screamed. I got to take my exams separately, received mostly A's and B's, and graduated *cum laude*.

"After working in human services for a while, I applied to and was accepted into a graduate social work program at a prestigious university. I did well and had one semester left before getting my master's degree when I was called into the dean's office. He said he did not feel I could function as a social worker because of the severity of my symptoms and thought that clinical placement wasn't possible for me. This, despite the fact that I had worked with clients and gotten along well with them and that my grades were excellent. I was devastated. I was obviously being discriminated against because of my TS.''

After having worked in the field for a few years, Joanne reapplied to the school, hoping to complete the remaining semester for her master's degree. She had gotten her medication under control and had lost more than a hundred pounds.

"The meeting focused on TS," she recalled bitterly. "They denied me readmittance, saying that I could not form empathetic relationships with clients and that I did not have the intellect to complete their program, although my test scores had all been extremely high. I felt that I had no recourse but to file an ADA federal lawsuit against them, which is now pending."

Joanne was then accepted into the Simmons School of Social Work in Boston, and, at this writing, received an A in her first course. She is on Risperdal and her speech is vastly improved from our first conversation. She reports that her tics are changing. They now are louder, but less intensive. She still has what she calls her, "nigger trigger," a tic that causes her to blurt out the racial slur when she sees a black person, but she is able to suppress it more now than before. "There was a black woman in my class and I didn't say it once all during the semester," she said proudly.

Joanne's advice?

- "Everyone in my neighborhood knows me so I've gotten pretty good at explaining what's wrong. I recommend your telling others about it. Learn to be comfortable telling others about what you have and what your needs are. Speak to the manager of stores you frequent. Become proactive.
- "Keep a sense of humor. It's helped me cope immeasurably. It eases tension in others and in yourself. Humor helps others to respond to me in a positive way.
- "Get special seating. I don't go to movies, but I do attend concerts and lectures. I ask for handicapped seating. I have an arm tic, so I ask for an empty seat next to me so I don't smash someone. Legally, they cannot charge you for the extra seat.

- "Know your rights about housing, employment, education, and so on. Know how to let people know *you* know your rights.
- "Don't have a chip on your shoulder. Have a good attitude."

"I avoid places where I'd be uncomfortable," she concluded. "If I go out to dinner, I'll go to tables around me and tell them what I have. Often they assume I'm deaf too because I'll hear them saying, 'Oh, Tourette Syndrome. I saw that on TV.' It's pretty rare that they haven't heard about it.

"The bottom line is gaining acceptance. People can't accept TS if they don't understand it. They can't understand it if they aren't educated about it. It's up to us to educate them."

Appendix A

Camps for Kids with TS

There are a number of camps, most of which are members of the American Camping Association, with programs for children with Tourette Syndrome. Contact the American Camping Association for their catalogue:

5000 State Road 67 North
Martinsville, IN 46151-7902
(317) 342-8456

Always get recommendations from other parents whose children have recently attended a particular camp. Also check with the Tourette Syndrome Association for the names of additional camps for children with TS.

Support Organizations

Tourette Syndrome Association
42–40 Bell Boulevard
Bayside, NY 11361–2874
(718) 224-2999
<tourette@ix.netcom.com>

They have the name and numbers of your nearest chapter as well as names of colleges with specialized programs for young people with TS, ADHD, and OCD; dentists, doctors, and so on. Call for a complete list of written and taped educational materials.

Children and Adults with Attention Deficit Disorders (CH.A.D.D.)

National Office

Children and Adults with Attention Deficit Disorders
499 N.W. 70th Avenue
Suite 101
Plantation, FL 33317
(305) 587-3700

There are more than five hundred of these groups located throughout the United States and Canada as well as on several military bases in Europe. The members meet once or twice a month with parents, adults with ADD, and health-care professionals to share information on medication, behavioral problems, and other specific issues relating to ADD. As the names of coordinators and their telephone numbers are subject to change, please call the national office for information concerning the chapter closest to you.

Learning Disabilities Association of America
4156 Library Road
Pittsburgh, PA 15234

This is the major parent organization on LD with chapters in most states.

OC Foundation

National Office

P.O. Box 70
Milford, CT 06460
(203) 878-5669
Fax: (203) 874-2826

There are OC groups located in almost all of the fifty states and in some Canadian provinces as well as in more than thirty foreign countries. Contact the national office for your nearest chapter.

American Association of Sex Educators, Counselors, and Therapists (AASECT)

Suite 1717
435 N. Michigan Avenue
Chicago, IL 60611

Equal Employment Opportunity Commission

1801 L Street, N.W.
Washington, DC 20507
(800) 669-EEOC

Alternative Therapy Network for Tourette Syndrome

P.O. Box 31256
Palm Beach Gardens, FL 33420-1256

Medic Alert

P.O. Box 1009
Turlock, CA 95381-1009
(800) 344-3226

Sibshop

Donald Meyer, Director of Sibling Support Project
Mail Stop C.L. 09
Children's Hospital and Medical Center
4800 Sand Point Way, N.E.
Seattle, WA 98105
(206) 368-4911

Those with computers and modems can communicate on-line with others interested in TS. CompuServe, Prodigy, America Online, and

Delphi all have TS forums. The address is Usnet: <alt.support. tourette>

CompuServe's TS group is found by first accessing the ADD forum. For Prodigy, jump "medical," and then select "neurological."

To learn how to arrange for your youngster to have special considerations, such as taking an untimed Scholastic Aptitude Test, write to the College Board, American Testing Program, Box 592, Princeton, NJ 08541.

Suggested Reading

Allen, Jeffrey G., J.D., C.P.C. *Successful Job Search Strategies for the Disabled* (New York, Chichester, Brisbane, Toronto, and Singapore: John Wiley & Sons, Inc., 1994).

Bain, Lisa J. *A Parent's Guide to Attention Deficit Disorders* (New York: Dell Trade Paperback, 1991).

Benson, Herbert, M.D., with Miriam Klipper. *The Relaxation Response* (New York: Avon Books, 1975).

Bolles, Richard Nelson. *The Three Boxes of Life* (Berkeley, CA: Ten Speed Press, 1981).

——————. *What Color Is Your Parachute?* (Berkeley, CA: Ten Speed Press, 1991).

Bruun, Ruth Dowling, M.D., and Bertel Bruun, M.D. *A Mind of Its Own: Tourette's Syndrome—A Story and a Guide* (New York: Oxford University Press, 1994).

Felder, Leonard, Ph.D. *When a Loved One Is Ill: How to Take Better Care of Your Loved One, Your Family, and Yourself* (New York: NAL Books, 1990).

Goldfarb, Lori A., Mary Jane Brotherson, Jean Ann Summers, and Ann P. Turnbull. *Meeting the Challenge of Disability or Chronic Illness—A Family Guide* (Baltimore: Paul H. Brookes Publishing Co., 1986).

Goldstein, Sam, and Michael Goldstein. *Hyperactivity: Why Won't My Child Pay Attention?* (New York: John Wiley & Sons, Inc., 1992).

Gordon, Sol. *When Living Hurts* (New York: Dell Publishing, 1985).

Haerle, Tracy. *Children with Tourette Syndrome* (Rockville, MD: Woodbine House, 1992).

Hallowell, Edward M., M.D., and John J. Ratey, M.D. *Driven to Distraction* (New York: Pantheon Books, 1994).

Kennedy, Patricia, Leif Terdal, Ph.D., and Lydia Fusetti, M.D. *The Hyperactive Child Book* (New York: St. Martin's Press, 1993).

Kushner, Harold S., Rabbi. *When Bad Things Happen to Good People* (New York: Avon, 1981).

McNamara, Barry E., Ed.D., and Francine J. McNamara, M.S.W., C.S.W. *Keys to Parenting a Child with Attention Deficit Disorder* (Hauppauge, NY: Barron's Educational Series, Inc., 1993).

Null, Gary. *No More Allergies* (New York: Villard Books, 1992).

Rapoport, Judith L., M.D. *The Boy Who Couldn't Stop Washing: The Experience and Treatment of Obsessive Compulsive Disease* (New York: Plume Books, 1989).

Rapp, Doris, M.D. *Is This Your Child?* (New York: William Morrow and Company, Inc., 1991).

Register, Cheri. *Living with Chronic Illness* (New York: Macmillan, Inc., 1987).

Sachs, Judith. *The Healing Power of Sex* (New York: Prentice Hall, 1994).

Sebastian, Richard. *The Encyclopedia of Health, Compulsive Behavior* (New York and Philadelphia: Chelsea House Publishers, 1993).

Silver, A. A., and R. A. Hagin. *Disorders of Learning in Childhood* (New York: John Wiley, 1990).

Silver, Larry B., M.D. *The Misunderstood Child: A Guide for Parents of Learning Disabled Children* (New York: TAB Books, 1992).

Steketee, G. S., and K. White. *When Once Is Not Enough* (Oakland, CA: New Harbinger Press, 1990).

Strong, Maggie. *Mainstay: For the Well Spouse of the Chronically Ill* (Boston: Little, Brown and Company, 1988).

Taylor, John F., Ph.D. *Helping Your Hyperactive Child* (Rocklin, CA: Prima Publishing & Communications, 1990).

Weiss, Gabrielle, and Lily Trokenberg Hechtman. *Hyperactive Children Grown Up* (New York: The Guilford Press, 1993).

Weiss, Lynn, Dr. *Attention Deficit Disorder in Adults* (Dallas: Taylor Publishing Company, 1992).

Glossary

Akathisia Inability to be still; a feeling of inner restlessness. It is a possible side effect of certain medications such as Haldol.

Antidepressant A prescription drug that relieves or minimizes depression.

Arithmomania Compulsive counting games.

Attention deficit hyperactivity disorder (ADHD) A neurological disorder which includes impulsive behavior, distractibility, and inability to focus attention.

Basal ganglia The specific interconnected groups of structures deep in the cerebral hemispheres of the brain and in the upper brainstem that relay messages between the front part of the brain and the lower motor and sensory areas.

Behavior therapy A type of therapy used with OCD and other conditions such as phobias, in which the person is exposed to anxiety-provoking stimuli while being prevented from performing the ritual or behavior previously used to reduce that anxiety.

CAT scan (also known as **CT scan**) Computerized axial tomography, a series of computerized X-rays of the brain.

Central nervous system (also known as **CNS**) Includes the brain and spinal cord.

Compulsion An overwhelming urge to perform a certain behavior in response to an obsession.

Coprolalia Involuntary utterances of obscene or inappropriate statements or words such as profanities.

Dopamine A chemical (neurotransmitter) in the brain.

Echolalia Repeating words or phrases of others.

Echopraxia Copying the gestures of others.

Etiology The cause of a disease.

Haloperidol (brand name **Haldol**) A medication used to treat TS.

Involuntary movements Actions that one cannot control.

Magnetic resonance imaging (also known as **MRI**) A scan of the brain or other part of the body which uses magnetic and low-energy radiowaves to produce x-ray–like pictures. However, no radioactive materials or dyes are used.

Monozygotic twins Identical twins.

Neurotransmitter Any of the chemicals carrying nerve impulses across the synapse (gap) between adjacent neurons (nerve cells).

Obsession An unwanted recurring idea, thought, image, or impulse that persists even though it makes no sense and the person tries to suppress it.

Obsessive-compulsive disorder (also known as **OCD**) An illness in which the person has uncontrollable thoughts and compulsive behavior to an extent that significantly impairs functioning.

Palilalia Repeating one's own words or phrases.

Positron emission tomography (also known as **PET**) An imaging technique using small amounts of radioactive material that produces a cross-sectional view of a type of chemical activity in the brain.

Premonitory urges Sensations immediately preceding an involuntary movement or vocalization (such as the sensations of one's nose tickling just before a sneeze).

Serotonin A chemical that acts as a neurotransmitter in the brain.

Synapse The gap between neurons, across which messages are carried by the chemicals called neurotransmitters.

Trichotillomania A compulsion to pull out one's hair in order to relieve anxiety.

Unvoluntary movements A term newly coined to reflect tics that one senses are coming, but can only suppress for a short period.

Index